Breast Cancer Surgery and Reconstruction

Breast Cancer Surgery and Reconstruction

What's Right for You

Patricia Anstett

with photography by Kathleen Galligan

ROWMAN & LITTLEFIELD
Lanham • Boulder • New York • London

Published by Rowman & Littlefield
A wholly owned subsidiary of The Rowman & Littlefield Publishing Group, Inc.
4501 Forbes Boulevard, Suite 200, Lanham, Maryland 20706
www.rowman.com

Unit A, Whitacre Mews, 26-34 Stannary Street, London SE11 4AB

British Library Cataloguing in Publication Information Available

Library of Congress Cataloging-in-Publication Data Available

ISBN: 978-1-4422-4262-3 (cloth : alk. paper)
eISBN: 978-1-4422-4263-0 (electronic)

♾™ The paper used in this publication meets the minimum requirements of
American National Standard for Information Sciences—Permanence of Paper
for Printed Library Materials, ANSI/NISO Z39.48-1992.

Printed in the United States of America

Contents

Acknowledgments   vii

Introduction   ix

1   Modern Breast Surgery and Reconstruction   1

2   Making the Decision   9

3   Mastectomy: What to Expect   19

4   A Veteran's Story: Lumpectomy   29

5   Reconstruction with Tissue   37

6   Medical Destinations   51

7   Silicone Implants   61

8   Saline Implants   73

9   Flat or One-Breasted   79

10   Uneven Results   93

11   Delayed Reconstruction   101

12   The Nipple: The Ultimate Challenge   111

13   Revisionists   119

14   Sex and Intimacy   127

15   Lymphedema   137

16   Arab Culture   145

17   Money and Insurance   155

18   Clothing and Breast Forms   163

19   Doctor Selection Issues   167

20   Previvors   177

21   Family   187

22   Pregnancy   201

23   Wrapping It Up   207

Notes   211

Glossary   217

Bibliography   223

Index   225

About the Author and Photographer   229

Acknowledgments

Patricia Anstett: This book could not have been done without: Donna Dauphinais, a friend who inspired this book with an invite to watch her nipple tattoo appointment; Canice Johnson, my high school writing teacher and mentor who died of breast cancer in May 2015; 240 donors who helped raise money for reporting and photography trips for the book; and my husband, Tim, and my children, Caitlin, Amy, and Eric, for whom I am eternally grateful for their love and support.

Kathleen Galligan: I express gratitude to the late Dawn Bhateley, an army friend who convinced me to tell my story; Bhateley died of breast cancer in September 2015; niece Erin Gallagher, photographer of my photo; Michelle Michalak, makeup and hair stylist; Seide Huschen, and Chris and Virginia Columbo of Columbo Scuba Adventures; Rachel Hessler, of Biker Bob's Harley-Davidson who loaned us her motorcycle for a photo session; to other women in this book who befriended me and supported me throughout my breast cancer treatment; and especially to my brother, John, and sister, Anne, who are always there for me.

Introduction

A modern era of breast cancer surgery and reconstruction has brought choices like never before for American women undergoing surgery to treat or prevent breast cancer.

But most don't emerge with new breasts and nipples in a single operation. It may take a year, even much longer, to finish the work, and complications can occur at any step along the way. Some never complete breast reconstruction, living without nipples or with breasts that don't match.

A growing trend toward double mastectomy and breast reconstruction in the United States, which raises concerns among many cancer experts, also threatens to overturn twenty-five years of public awareness about the success of lumpectomy and radiation for treating most early-stage breast cancers.

Breast Cancer Surgery and Reconstruction: What's Right for You reframes the important discussion about lumpectomy, mastectomy, and breast reconstruction around the women who have had these operations. It offers women's unique viewpoints about the less discussed but essential part of breast cancer: the surgery nearly every woman has, regardless of whether she has reconstruction or not.

1

Modern Breast Surgery and Reconstruction

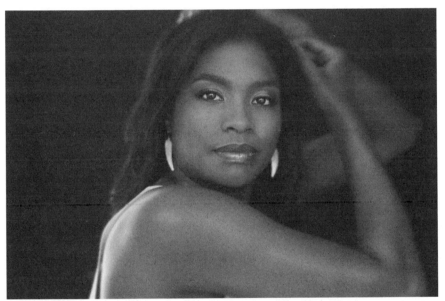

Cheryl Perkins was thirty-five, nursing her fourth child, when she found out she had breast cancer.

Cheryl Perkins was just thirty-five, nursing her fourth child, when she found out she had breast cancer. She had three other young daughters and a full-time job as a registered nurse in Detroit.

Her obstetrician assured her the lump she found probably was a clogged milk duct, but Perkins persisted and got a mammogram. The test found an aggressive tumor that had spread under her armpit. It was a stage 2, triple-negative breast cancer, a type of tumor that doesn't respond well to standard chemotherapies because it lacks cell receptors that drugs target for estrogen and progesterone hormones and a protein called HER2/neu.

For reasons not yet understood, triple-negative tumors are more common in women who are young, black, or who carry mutations for two known BRCA1 and BRCA2 genes.

Perkins had a life to get on with and fears to put at rest as best as she could. She asked her hairdresser to trim her shoulder-length hair to a short, Halle Berry cut and told her kids, "I'm going to fight this." She had a double mastectomy with immediate reconstruction with saline implants, a decision she made quickly, with her gut instincts, even though she's a registered nurse.

"When I found out I had cancer on the right side I wanted to eliminate the risk it would happen on the left," she recalled. "I wanted to feel a little more at ease, to have some kind of peace of mind. I wanted to be sure it didn't come back."

In a new era of breast cancer surgery and reconstruction, young and middle-aged women like Perkins with breast cancer, as well as women with gene mutations that greatly raise their risk of getting breast cancer, are changing the discussion as never before.

Some bring surgery preferences, including double mastectomy; more aggressive styles of selecting physicians; and other issues, from fertility to hormone replacement therapy, that are likely to have a profound influence for years on breast cancer surgery and reconstruction in the United States.

Though breast cancer remains largely a disease of aging, with the risk of getting it increasing as a woman gets older, the demographics of women undergoing surgery and reconstruction have changed drastically in just the last few years.

An announcement in 2013 by actress Angelina Jolie[1] that she underwent preventive nipple-sparing double mastectomy with silicone reconstruction only heightened public awareness and interest in genetic counseling and preventive surgeries, particularly among young women, even teenagers. Cancer centers called it the Angelina effect; some women even asked to be tested for the Angelina gene.

The same year of Jolie's surgery, Kelly Rothe became one of the youngest known women in the United States to have preventive surgery. Rothe, twenty, a college junior at the time, had to convince her breast surgeon she was mature enough to understand the implications of her decision to have a double mastectomy.

Emmy Pontz-Rickert was twenty-four when she had a double mastectomy and chemotherapy for an aggressive tumor. She gave birth to her first child, Grace, in 2015. She regrets being unable to breastfeed her daughter but is thrilled to be a mother, particularly given what she went through just two years earlier.

Sara Erzen was thirty-five, pregnant with her third child, when she found a lump in her breast that was cancerous. She completed her surgery and reconstruction only to develop an infection in the expander phase of the procedure. She lives one-breasted. For now, reconstruction isn't important.

These days, entire families make surgery decisions together, like Alejandra Rojas, sixty-three, of Santa Ana, California, and three of her four daughters, ages twenty-nine to thirty-five, who carry BRCA1 gene mutations. They and others travel to national meetings of women with hereditary syndromes to hear top cancer surgeons. Or they schedule procedures at out-of-town medical destinations catering to women looking for the best.

You will meet these women and others interested in passing on lessons learned from their own breast cancer surgery and reconstruction decisions. We found them through breast cancer organizations, physicians and specialists, friends, and professional contacts. They agreed to be interviewed and photographed, and some even allowed us to watch their surgery and reconstruction procedures or let us follow them for updates. We also interviewed some of the top breast and plastic surgeons and obtained rare privileges to watch entire procedures, including lumpectomy, mastectomy, fat grafting, and dermal injections, several types of breast reconstruction, and nipple tattooing. What emerges from two years of reporting across the country is a completely different approach to an important but underdiscussed breast cancer issue, told in moving, real stories with women you will connect with, along with interviews with experts about the most important issues. We hope to bring women new resources and give doctors a fresh, new approach to talking about breast cancer surgery and reconstruction with their patients.

Today, women have better choices than ever before, including new approaches—such as breast reconstruction with a woman's own tissue and nipple-sparing mastectomy.

Over the last decade, implant reconstruction also has improved with fat-grafting methods and acellular dermal matrix products made from sterilized human and pig collagen used to add support and shape around an implant.

Implants themselves continue to evolve, including larger sizes for bigger-breasted, plus-sized, and larger-framed women. In the past, busty or large women had to settle for smaller breasts because larger implants were unavailable in the United States.

Equally important, many women now have a way to pay for breast reconstruction. Since 1998, a federal law has required most health plans to pay for reconstruction or breast forms after mastectomy.[2]

In 2015, a ruling by the Obama administration also said insurers must pay for preventive surgeries, as well as genetic counseling and testing, for high-risk women, according to a May 11, 2015, *New York Times* story by health reporter Robert Pear.

With choices like these, interest in reconstruction and breast revision is strong and likely to increase for years, particularly as more young women have preventive surgeries.

The changes and advances obscure one important reality: most American women never undergo reconstruction, and many don't need to.

More than 230,000 women were estimated to be diagnosed with breast cancer in the United States in 2014, according to the American Cancer Society. About 60 percent or 138,000 of those women have a breast-sparing lumpectomy and radiation, large studies suggest.[3]

That compares to 102,215 breast reconstruction procedures,[4] often performed after a double mastectomy.

A 2014 study of national cancer registry data from Los Angeles and Detroit gave new perspectives on why women diagnosed with breast cancer declined reconstruction.[5] Most didn't want it, and still didn't, four years later. The most common reasons women gave for declining reconstruction were:

- desire to avoid additional surgery, 48.5 percent
- reconstruction wasn't important, 33.8 percent
- fear of implants, 36.3 percent

"If there's one message from the study, it's there is not a big problem here," said Dr. Monica Morrow, chief breast surgeon at Memorial Sloan Kettering Cancer Center in New York and lead author. "The vast majority were very happy with their decision and the information they received four years later."

Another emerging trend, however, concerns Morrow and many other top cancer doctors.

Although 70 to 90 percent of women have breast cancers that can be treated with lumpectomy and radiation, only about 60 percent of women do, studies show. Increasingly, women are choosing to have a double mastectomy even when they do not have cancer in both breasts.[6] Experts worry that the trend will overturn more than two decades of public awareness about the value of lumpectomy. Consensus guidelines issued in 1990 cited studies that women lived just as long with a lumpectomy and radiation as they did after a mastectomy.[7]

In 2014, two leading cancer organizations issued new consensus guidelines clarifying the role of lumpectomy in early-stage breast cancer. The goal was to decrease the number of women who undergo more than one lumpectomy because of the lack of "clear margins"—cancer-free areas around the lump that was removed.

Because women also receive radiation, additional lumpectomy surgery, or reexcisions, should not be necessary most of the time, the guidelines said.[8]

"We need to help women understand that radiation is there to do the job picking up any cancer left behind," Morrow said. "We want women to have the confidence to select a lumpectomy rather than a mastectomy when medically possible and breast cancer physicians to be confident about knowing when a margin is adequate."

The guidelines address the fact that one in four women undergoing lumpectomy returned for at least one more surgery, only to find half the time there was no sign of cancer in the margins of the tumor. Reexcision rates varied widely among doctors, from 0 percent to as much as 70 percent, the research found.

———————————

Looking back, whether a woman has breast-sparing surgery or a mastectomy with reconstruction, many mention a list of things they wish they had known before breast cancer surgery. Even the most educated women find recovery after mastectomy, with or without reconstruction, surprisingly more challenging than they thought.

Women say they underestimated the impact of surgery or felt poorly prepared to handle problems, including implant and expander issues that sent them to the hospital. Others say they needed more time to recover than they expected.

"I really didn't understand that the reconstruction process was going to be so painful," said Judith Medeiros Fitzgerald, a retired Portsmouth, Rhode Island, teacher diagnosed with cancer in both of her breasts in 2009. She had a bilateral mastectomy with implant reconstruction using expanders. "After surgery, it basically hurt to breathe," she said. "I couldn't sleep well. I'd have to put pillows under my arms and arm movement was very limited. They finally prescribed physical therapy, which a lot of women aren't advised is available."

Fitzgerald wonders how much she heard but didn't fully process. "Maybe I didn't want to know it would be rough. I had my mind so made up. I wanted the cancer gone. I honestly wasn't prepared for six months of extremely limited mobility and lymphedema on my left side," she said of chronic arm pain she developed.

Fitzgerald's experience became a journal, then a book, *A Teacher's Journey . . . What Breast Cancer Taught Me.*[9] It also triggered her interest in a different direction, to the prevention of breast cancer. She informs and lobbies for money for breast cancer vaccine research on her organization's website, http://www.sisters4prevention.com. Her hope is that surgery someday may not be necessary, at least for some. Phase One trials of a vaccine could begin as early as 2016, she said.

Jill Courson, forty-nine, an audiologist and mother of two boys, twenty and eighteen, highly recommends having a support team in place to help in the months during and after surgery or treatment. She created a Facebook page about her cancer treatment throughout 2012 to 2014 that kept friends and family updated about her progress. "I had about 25 of my best friends and my siblings who were able to check on me instead of making phone calls," she said. "My sister-in-law posted what was going on, even during my 13-hour mastectomy surgery. It was great going and seeing what all my girlfriends would say. One group was in Cancun at the time and they posted on my Facebook a toast to me. I did the same thing, only I had my Styrofoam water cup. I thought it was good for my sons to see so many people being so supportive."

Friends arranged meal trains. "That was awesome. My youngest son really looked forward to the meal train. It came every other week for three days, after chemo."

Courson, who had divorced ten months before her diagnosis, said she is glad that she let her girlfriends "take over."

"I have a really close network of girlfriends and they were just amazing," said Courson, who lives in Grosse Pointe, Michigan. "They attended all my doctors' appointments and my surgeries. I think what I did very well was gather my team members without whom I would not have been successful. I did continue to work. I would suggest that. It wasn't easy at all but it was very helpful to wake up every morning and go somewhere. I took eight weeks off of work, six for the mastectomy and two for the exchange."

Courson, an athlete who was parasailing and zip-lining several months after her surgeries, advises women not to hesitate communicating strong feelings and intentions to their doctors.

"I gave them very strict instructions," she said. "I play sports. I'm very active. I ride a bike. I've played volleyball my entire life. I play tennis. I didn't want them to be touching in the middle. I didn't want to have anything falling down on the sides and I didn't want them to be bigger than what I had before. One of the reasons I kept my areolas was because they are above average in size and if they took those too, my breasts would be smaller than what I used to have."

Courson developed bleeding from a hematoma in the exchange portion of her implant surgery. "After my exchange, when they took the expander out and put the implants in, one of the breasts got real swollen and painful. I had to have emergency surgery to reopen the incision and take out the implant and suction out the blood. The pain medicine made me vomit so much that I was told I ripped a pec muscle and it was bleeding and filling up the pocket where the implant was. They had to cauterize the muscle, clean it up and put another implant back in. Thankfully, I had told a friend she could spend the night and she was there to help when it happened."

Courson took pictures along the way, including some that were jarring to her friends. "My girlfriends would get freaked out because they thought for sure that my nipples would end up underneath my armpits," she said. "They said, 'I can't believe you didn't get upset.' I said, 'Why should I get upset about anything? There's nothing I can do about it. I just have to wait until everything comes out right.'"

And it did.

In 2015, she traveled abroad with her sons, played on volleyball and tennis teams, and looked forward to a year with no cancer treatment.

———————

Twelve years after her double mastectomy and reconstruction, Cheryl Perkins, now a neonatal nurse, wonders if she'll go back for more.

She lived with her first set of saline implants for seven years until one got hard and infected. They were replaced with silicone implants, which "worked well," particularly because she has some damage from radiation, she said.

Radiation darkened and thinned her skin and gave her a bust line that is "more barrel-shaped," she said. "They are not what I expected them to be," she said. "I was hoping for C cups or something big so I could look really va-va-voom," said Perkins. "That never worked out because my skin was too tight from radiation." Her plastic surgeon also blamed radiation for the failure of one of two nipples he made for her with fat grafts and dermal filler material.

Perkins still may return for another try at a nipple. She's recently divorced, and she wonders how others might react to her unmatched breasts. "I thought my husband accepted me the way they were, only to find out not really," she said. "Being in the marketplace, looking for a mate, I'm concerned how that is going to go over and whether someone would be weirded out by it."

She overcame some of her inhibitions as a ballroom dancer in a Dancing with the Survivors® fund-raiser event in October 2014 in Bloomfield Hills, Michigan, for The Pink Fund, a nonprofit that gives up to $3,000 in help paying nonmedical bills for women currently undergoing breast cancer treatment. The year before, she was chosen to be one of the breast cancer survivor models for a Ford Motor Company Warriors in Pink campaign, which has raised $128 million for breast cancer groups, including The Pink Fund.[10]

Overall, she has gotten past the cancer diagnosis that seemed to frame her life for too long.

"My advice is, be patient with it. Realize you will be a new you. You just have to come to grips with your new look. You'll feel fine. You'll feel womanly again. It just takes time. I guess with cancer, you're not sure how much time you have to deal with this. It's definitely a question to wonder: Is it worth it? How much time do I have on earth? Is it that important to me to have the appearances of a woman? I was 35 when diagnosed. It was important to me to look normal."

2

Making the Decision

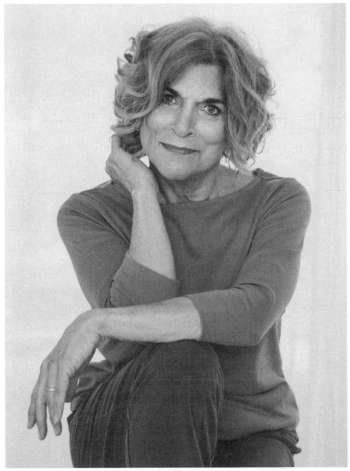

Sharon Kiley Heck is one of a growing number of American women undergoing double mastectomies, even though they only have cancer in one breast.

With a mother and sister diagnosed with breast cancer, Sharon Kiley Heck always was vigilant about getting mammograms and doing self-exams.

A month after she got a mammogram with no sign of cancer, she found a pea-sized lump in her left breast.

Her doctors told her that she had a lobular tumor "more likely to go to the other breast," recalled Heck, seventy, of Fort Wright, Kentucky, a suburb of Cincinnati. She also needed chemotherapy.

She chose to have a double mastectomy with silicone breast reconstruction. Her decision was based on her family's cancer history and her new life as wife and stepmother to three children whose mother had died. She reasoned that a double mastectomy would best ensure that her kids didn't have to lose another mother. "I raised them; I was their mom. I didn't want them to go through that again."

More than twenty-four years later, she still has the same implants and is pleased with her choice. More importantly, she has lived life without the constant fear of a cancer recurrence.

"I just didn't want the hammer hanging over me anymore," explained Heck, a retired GE Aviation human resource specialist. "I wanted to be rid of it, to make sure I wasn't going to have a recurrence or anything."

Heck, who had her surgery in January 1991, was among the last American women to get silicone breast implants outside of a research study in the United States for the next sixteen years. A year later, the federal Food and Drug Administration imposed a ban on silicone implants because of safety issues. It was lifted in November 2006 when implant manufacturers gave the agency data showing silicone implants were safe.[1]

The increase in contralateral prophylactic mastectomy, as surgery to remove a noncancerous breast is called, is one of the most significant women's health developments in several decades.

At a time when as much as 70 to 90 percent of all women with early-stage 1 and 2 tumors are candidates for lumpectomy, more women like Heck are choosing to have bilateral mastectomy procedures to remove both breasts after a cancer diagnosis, even though they only have cancer in one breast. The fear of the cancer's return, along with the hope of having matching breasts, have become powerful factors in a woman's choice of a double mastectomy instead of lumpectomy. Others pick mastectomy because of concerns about radiation and the six-to-eight weeks of daily treatments it requires.

Women with early-stage breast cancers who underwent double mastectomies increased from 34.3 percent in 1998 to 37.8 percent in 2011, one large study published in 2014 found.[2] Of concern to experts: women who opted for double mastectomy the most had no positive lymph nodes and noninvasive cancers, such as ductal carcinoma in situ.

The trend threatens to undo more than two decades of public aware-ness about the value of lumpectomy and radiation. Lucette Lagnado's *Wall Street Journal* story on July 13, 2015, went as far as to dub it "The Mastectomy Rebellion." Others call the extra surgery unnecessary or troubling.

"It's a little disturbing and it bears watching," said Dr. Allen Lichter, a radiation oncologist who helped conduct the landmark studies that led to 1990 national consensus guidelines reinforcing the equal survival ben-efits of lumpectomy and radiation in early-stage breast cancer treatment compared to mastectomy.[3]

"I certainly understand the motivation, at a certain level," said Lichter, chief executive officer of the American Society of Clinical Oncology, a leading cancer research organization. "Clearly a double mastectomy has finality to it. It brings some peace of mind. However, it's challenging to take a normal body part as a preventive intervention for something that is relatively low risk. There's not much precedent to take another body part but it's become fairly common in breast cancer. It's not like taking out a kidney or a lung."

"Certainly women who have mutations that put them at an enormously high risk of breast cancer are in a different category. But for the average woman the risk of a contralateral breast cancer is probably in the range of a few percent. And there are other factors: the need for continued surveil-lance; the anxiety of the annual mammogram and the potential callback for a biopsy. There is a host of consequences of leaving that breast for some women. As they weigh the small risk of getting cancer, all that ends up tipping the scale."

Guidelines from the National Comprehensive Cancer Network, a group of top academic cancer centers, discourage contralateral prophy-lactic mastectomy unless a woman carries a gene mutation that raises her risk, which is about 5 to 10 percent of all breast cancers. Otherwise, the extra surgery offers no extra survival benefit, the guidelines say.[4]

Studies published more recently show an even stronger survival ad-vantage for women undergoing lumpectomy and radiation, said Diana Zuckerman, PhD, president of the National Center for Health Research and founder of its Cancer Prevention and Treatment Fund, a Washington, D.C., nonprofit organization. The organization has a free helpline, patient booklets, and Zuckerman's reviews of breast surgery and implants, avail-able through its http://www.stopcancerfund.org website.

"This fear of breast cancer is out of proportion to reality," said Zucker-man, a widely published scientist whose research about the lack of safety data led to congressional hearings and soon a federal moratorium on silicone implants in 1992.

"Heart disease is the number-one killer of women," Zuckerman said. "Why is it we are so afraid of breast cancer? Women understandably fear getting a disease that will cause them to get their breasts removed, so why do so many deal with that fear by having their breasts removed when it isn't medically necessary?"

Zuckerman pointed to research showing that women with early-stage breast cancer have a slightly better survival rate when they have a lumpectomy than a mastectomy. She also described a very large August 2015 study that found that women with stage 0 breast cancer known as ductal carcinoma in situ, DCIS, have almost identical odds of dying of breast cancer as women in the general population—3 percent compared to 1.5 percent.[5]

Research also shows that if more doctors called DCIS a lesion instead of cancer, women are less likely to have a healthy breast removed, she said.

"Experts now agree that most of these breast abnormalities would never become cancer, even if they were not treated," explained Zucker-man. "What is the big rush to remove breasts at the first sign of any abnormality, and how can we help a woman with early-stage breast cancer realize that removing her breast will not have a positive impact on her health? That's a very big question. Part of the answer might be to be more precise about using the term cancer only when the condition really is a cancer that is capable of spreading at some point in the future. We need to do a better job of talking to patients so that they are not unduly frightened."

Given the debate, women and doctors may spend time at their first preoperative appointment discussing research put into a risk-versus-benefit approach.

"We want women to understand that having the bilateral or double mastectomy doesn't increase the chances of beating that first cancer," said Dr. Lisa Newman, director of the breast oncology program for the Henry Ford Health System in Detroit, Michigan. "We want them to understand they are not gaining a survival advantage by undergoing a double mastectomy and that the medical or systemic treatment for the initially-diagnosed breast cancer, such as recommendations for chemotherapy, will be the same regardless of whether she has a single or double mastectomy," she said.

"We never want a patient to choose to undergo contralateral prophylactic mastectomy because of the incorrect perception that it will take away the need for chemotherapy, or that it reduces the chances of the known cancer recurring on the chest wall or metastasizing to other organs of the body," Newman added. "Once the patient understands that preventive surgery is not a medical necessity, that it does not affect the success rate for treatment of the known, first cancer, and that it does not completely eliminate the possibility of getting a new, second breast cancer, then it really becomes a personal judgment call for the patient."

"We have to tell women what their risks are and what their survival rates are. We counsel them about their safest cancer treatment options but beyond that it's a woman's choice to decide whether prevention surgery is worthwhile."

In the end, it's a patient's decision, Newman said. "If a breast cancer patient says that she's losing sleep worrying about the risk of developing a new cancer within a remaining breast on her chest wall, or if she says she wants to do whatever she can to minimize the possibility of having to repeat the breast cancer diagnosis and treatment experience again, such as going through chemotherapy or having to undergo lymph node surgery for a new breast cancer, then prophylactic contralateral mastectomy may in fact be a reasonable choice for her."

"I think it's wrong for us to be dogmatic with patients. We have an obligation to explain the safe and appropriate cancer treatment options, but we have to then respect the patient's decision."

Dr. Edwin Wilkins, professor of plastic surgery at the University of Michigan, Ann Arbor, added, "Women often know better than I do what's going to work best for them. Our jobs as researchers and clinicians are to gather the information that's relevant and timely and pass that along to patients in a format that lets them make the best decision. The answer is different for different people, even by ethnicity and race, which is something we are looking at."

Wilkins is the principal investigator of the Mastectomy Reconstruction Outcomes Consortium (MROC) Study, one of the largest ever conducted. It is following three thousand women throughout the country at ten large North American cancer centers to measure patient satisfaction and other issues with breast cancer surgery and reconstruction. Its findings are expected by 2016, though some research has been published already.[6] The new study, an extension of an earlier arm of the study completed in 1998, will examine several new issues, including postoperative pain, fatigue, and depression after breast cancer surgery, he said.

"Patients want to know how soon they will feel back to normal," Wilkins said. "One of the things we found early on is that these operations take longer to recover from than we thought. That's different than what we had been telling people, that a month or two after the surgery they'd be pretty much back to normal. It turns out that people are mostly back to normal most of the time—but not completely. Even at three months out, they are not quite back up to their normal energy levels. When people plan to have these operations and weigh how they affect their daily lives, they need to know these things."

Wilkins said he was surprised by early findings of the latest study to see high rates of depression, anxiety, and even thoughts of suicide in women having breast cancer surgery and reconstruction.

"We found with immediate reconstruction that newly diagnosed breast cancer patients had rates of moderate to severe depression of around 15–17%. About the same proportion had clinically diagnosable anxiety disorders. The other thing we found early on was that about one patient out of 100 was engaged in active suicidal ideation. These are much more emotionally traumatized people than I would have suspected, having dealt with them for 30 years."

The University of Michigan is designing a way to reach out to women participating in the survey who express suicidal thoughts or who have anxiety or depression so they can find help easily if needed, he said. Even a year or two after surgery, women's emotions, feelings about body image, and satisfaction with their surgery may change. Fortunately, most women eventually feel good about their choice and their outcomes, he said.

"The most striking thing from our early study in the 1990s was that the type of breast reconstruction—implants or flaps—didn't matter as much as we as surgeons thought it would," Wilkins said. "Instead, what turned out to matter the most was that people who needed and wanted reconstruction got it and reaped the rewards in terms of quality of life. If there is a single central finding from the old study that was it."

———————⸎———————

The decision about what type of breast surgery to have and whether to undergo breast reconstruction is a highly personal one.

The type of cancer a woman has, the size and location in the breast of a tumor, a woman's weight and breast size all are factors that can influence surgery choices.

Research studies cite other factors that affect surgery decisions, including a woman's doctors and hospital, and whether they perform breast reconstruction; where she lives; whether she works or has family responsibilities; her education and income; and travel times to radiation facilities in urban areas.

One large review published in 2015 found that lumpectomy and radiation was preferred among women fifty-two to sixty-one years of age, along with those who had higher income levels, comprehensive health insurance, were treated at a university-affiliated hospital, and lived within seventeen miles of a radiation facility.[7]

"For a lot of women there's a sense that I need to get this over with," Zuckerman said. They feel they can't take time off of work so they think radiation is not going to be an option, either because of work or geographic isolation from a radiation facility. I think this one decision leads to another. Maybe it's partly because we live in a society where you feel you can't take four weeks off from work or from taking care of your family. But they will usually need to take more time off later if they undergo a mastectomy with reconstruction now."

Women who need chemotherapy for more aggressive tumors must decide how surgery can be timed with other therapies, said Dr. Michael Meininger, a Beaumont Hospital, Royal Oak, Michigan, plastic surgeon.

"I'll start by explaining I'm a breast preservationist by nature," Meininger said. "If that opposite breast is not a liability to you, then you are best keeping it. It's a normal breast. It feels normal. It looks normal. It has a nipple. It has normal sensations. We should work with trying to make your reconstructed breast as much like your normal breast as we can. And if we can't, we alter the other breast to make it match."

"The other approach we take is what is called a risk and benefit analysis. Everything we do in surgery has a risk. There could be bleeding or infection, a pneumonia or a urinary tract infection, a clot, wound-healing problems, you name it. My big fear with doing elective reconstruction at the time of a mastectomy is that my surgery is going to cause a complication that will result in a delay in treatment. They've got to do their chemotherapy or radiation in a month to six weeks. You do a prophylactic mastectomy and an infection occurs. That takes 10 days to develop and it takes another 10 days for you to successfully treat it. It takes another two weeks to completely heal. Then you've delayed their treatment by a month to a month and a half. Then, I've hurt her. First do no harm. It goes right down to that."

—————«(•)»—————

Sharon Kiley Heck feels she made the right decision. Her cancer diagnosis was a "bigger deal" than removing a noncancerous breast, she said.

"Problems? Never," said Heck. "My expectation is I won't have to have them replaced. It's been more than 24 years. If they haven't leaked or whatever by now, I don't think they are going to. There is a lot of scar tissue around them by now so I think they are well set."

Heck's reconstructed breasts sit higher on her chest, and "they really are larger than I would hope for them to be. I don't think they look anything like breasts. They look like little skin-colored bowls that sit where my breasts would be. I never got tattooed. I just wanted the nipples so I didn't have a bare chest, which would look very unusual to me. So I went ahead and got the nipples," with extra skin moved to her chest and wrapped to create a new pair.

"I also had no idea I'd lose all feeling in my chest. No one ever mentioned that to me, which I would have appreciated if they had, so I would have gotten used to the idea. I only had been married for three years at the time and my husband and I were at a pretty deep stage of our sex lives. But that didn't stop."

Still, when she goes to bed at night, "I turn out the light and climb in under the covers. I also turn my back when I get undressed. I'm so shy that no one except my husband has seen me naked since my surgery. And he doesn't get as much of that as he'd like. Fortunately, I have a very healthy sex drive, which wasn't dimmed by the surgery."

Heck's breasts cause her "occasional discomfort just because there's a foreign body and it moves around and gets into a funny place where I kind of have to tweak it around a little bit to get it to where it's supposed to be." Plastic surgeons call this movement "distortion."

Sometimes, "I have this tightness around my chest, like a band around my upper body," Heck said. "It's never gone away. I worry that when I hug someone they're going to think I will feel funny, although no one has ever said that."

Heck understands that the tightness may be a sign of an implant problem, such as capsular contracture, but has chosen to live with it. It causes her no other symptoms, and it's not a problem to her, she said.

Women also need to know it may take a year before their new breasts settle in, she said.

"It took a while to get my wardrobe in shape and I wore bras for several years. I probably needed one in the beginning after reconstruction. But at some point my physiology in my chest became so stable that the implants stopped moving around and I stopped wearing bras."

"I don't even own one now. It's been a long time since I have worn a bra."

MORE HELP

For more help, visit the National Cancer Institute at www.cancer.gov/cancertopics/pdq/treatment/breast/healthprofessional/Page6#Section_437. It lists guidelines for breast cancer based on tumor characteristics and other factors.

The NCI also has prepared a list of questions to ask doctors to help make breast cancer surgery decisions. They include:

- What are my treatment choices? Which do you recommend for me? Why?
- What are the expected benefits and risks of the treatment?
- What can I do to prepare for treatment?
- Will I need to stay in the hospital? If so, for how long?

- What is the treatment likely to cost? Will my insurance cover it?
- How will treatment affect my normal activities?
- Would a research study, also called a clinical trial, be right for me?
- If I decide to have plastic surgery to rebuild my breast, how and when can that be done?
- Can you suggest a plastic surgeon for me to contact?

The National Comprehensive Cancer Network, a national coalition of cancer organizations, also has helpful resources on its site, www .nccn.org/patients/guidelines/.

Others recommend bringing a second person, or a tape recorder, to make sure you understand the information presented. If a doctor is uncomfortable with such a request, find someone else, many experts say. Also, ask a plastic surgeon if the plastic surgery she primarily performs is implant reconstruction or tissue-based procedures as well. The success of these surgeries is closely related to the amount of experience of the surgeon doing them.

3
Mastectomy: What to Expect

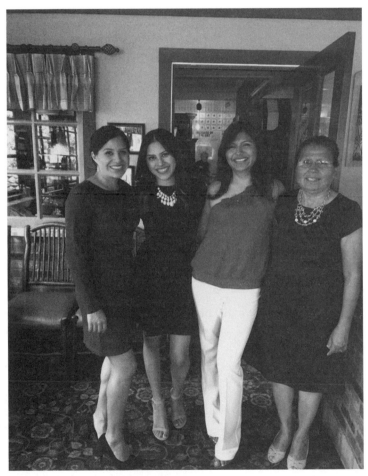

Veronica Rojas-Gudino, second from right, is one of three sisters having preventive surgery or close monitoring of cancer because they carry a gene mutation. Photo from Rojas family.

For a person ready to have both of her breasts removed, even though she didn't have cancer, Veronica Rojas-Gudino looked quite calm.

She has thought carefully about her decision for nearly four years.

Now, Rojas-Gudino, thirty-five, a Santa Ana, California teacher, was ready to move ahead with the last stage of her plan to try to never have cancer.

She was having a preventive, nipple-sparing double mastectomy with silicone implant reconstruction. Because she is healthy, young, and has no cancer, Rojas-Gudino was an ideal candidate for the operation. In fact, her surgeon, Dr. Michele Carpenter of St. Joseph Hospital in Orange, California, was so pleased with how smoothly it went that she called it "a textbook mastectomy."

No other surgery than nipple-sparing mastectomy epitomizes the modern era of breast reconstruction in the United States.

It has been around for more than a decade, but interest in it has been high since 2013, when actress Angelina Jolie said she had a preventive, bilateral, nipple-sparing mastectomy with silicone implant reconstruction.[1]

Nipple-sparing mastectomy saves a woman's nipple and areola, improving the final appearance of the breast and avoiding the potentially troublesome construction of a new nipple and areola.

A skin-sparing mastectomy, by comparison, saves all of the outer breast skin except the nipple and areola; it usually is done when cancer is nearby.

Today, surgeons like Carpenter see nearly as many women without cancer asking them about nipple-sparing operations as women with cancer.

By having a double mastectomy, Rojas-Gudino lowered her risk of getting breast cancer by as much as 90 percent, according to the National Cancer Institute.[2] She reduced her chance of getting ovarian cancer by 50 percent with a hysterectomy and removal of her ovaries and fallopian tubes in December 2014.

"I really wanted to have a girl but it didn't happen," said Rojas-Gudino, who has two boys, five and ten. "My husband said it's best to take care of yourself."

Rojas-Gudino and two of three sisters and their mother have the BRCA1 mutation that raises their risk significantly of getting breast or ovarian cancer. Veronica's mother, Alejandra, was diagnosed before age sixty with both breast and ovarian cancer, three years apart. A younger sister, Socorro, already has had both preventive surgeries, and a third, Erika, is pregnant and watching her cancer risk with tests.

<hr>

Nipple-sparing operations are one of several types of modern mastectomy procedures.

ELIGIBILITY FOR NIPPLE-SPARING MASTECTOMY

Can most women have a nipple-sparing mastectomy?

Many younger women, and most without cancer, are good candidates, doctors say.

Many quickly add: the smaller the breast, the better.

"Women with A-cup, B-cup breasts, you can pretty much guarantee great results," said Dr. Scott Karlan, a Los Angeles plastic surgeon addressing the annual meeting in June 2015 of Facing Our Risk of Cancer Empowered (FORCE), a national nonprofit organization of women with hereditary cancer risks. "Very rarely do you run into blood supply issues to the nipple."

For other women, particularly those with large or droopy breasts, there is a greater risk the nipple will not survive, he said. "Some people are just poor candidates and that probably should be recognized and they should be told that up front."

Women diagnosed with cancer also may be eligible for nipple-sparing mastectomy if their tumors are not too large or located near the nipple and they have not had prior radiation.

Dr. Andrew Ashikari, a Dobbs Ferry, New York, plastic surgeon who was one of the first to offer nipple-sparing mastectomy in the United States, said that while women with large or droopy breasts "are tougher cases," they, too, can have the procedure, although a revision surgery such as a breast lift might be needed. He also was at the FORCE conference in a Q&A panel on breast cancer surgery.

The American Society of Breast Surgeons has created a registry that will track survival, patient satisfaction, and other outcomes from a large group of participating institutions. But results aren't expected for several years.

Until then, enough concerns remain that the American Cancer Society warned in a March 12, 2015, medical review: "Nipple-sparing operations have some problems. Afterward, the nipple does not have a good blood supply, so sometimes it can wither away or become deformed. Because the nerves are also cut, there's little or no feeling in the nipple. In some cases, the nipple may look out of place later, mostly in women with larger breasts. Doctors are working to improve the safety and outcomes of nipple-sparing surgeries."

Several studies have concluded the technique is successful and safe. "Our review demonstrates that nipple-sparing mastectomy and immediate reconstruction has a high rate of success and a low rate of complications," wrote Dr. Amy S. Colwell, a breast surgeon at Massachusetts General Hospital, Boston, in a March 4, 2014, press release from the American Society of Plastic Surgeons, which published the research.

The most common types of mastectomy are a total mastectomy, also called a simple mastectomy, in which no lymph nodes under the arm are removed; it is performed in 45 percent of mastectomy surgeries; and a modified radical mastectomy, which removes some lymph nodes, which is done 34.7 percent of the time, according to one large study cited on breastcancer.org, a popular site with extensive resources.[3]

Less commonly used, a partial mastectomy removes slightly more tissue than a breast-sparing lumpectomy. A radical mastectomy, now rarely done, removes breast tissue, some lymph nodes, and underlying muscle.

Mastectomy operations with implant reconstruction are quite similar. Women live with surgical drains in their chest for a week to ten days to remove fluid, a rigorous, often annoying phase of recovery. Hospitals also follow strict standards for anesthesia, airway management, instrument accountability, and other issues in an era of patient safety.

Before surgery, patients get a list of instructions to follow and medications to stop. They are encouraged to stop smoking, if they do. Patients stay as little as a day, like Rojas-Gudino, or up to three days, typically, for mastectomy with implant reconstruction.

Rojas-Gudino and her husband, Victor, reported for check-in at 12:15 p.m. on July 30, 2015. As instructed, she wore no jewelry; hadn't eaten since midnight; and she showered with an antibacterial soap, her last full shower for at least a week.

Rojas-Gudino came to the operation fully informed. She had genetics counseling. She carefully followed cancer-screening recommendations such as annual mammograms while she made up her mind. And she and two sisters went so far as to attend two national conferences of FORCE.

She made arrangements with her mom to watch her two boys for the night. "I want her to be safe in the future," said Victor, her husband of eleven years, explaining his support for her decisions to have preventive surgery. She hoped for a quick recovery and to have reconstruction fully completed by November, when she has some time off work. She knows an infection or any problem will delay her plans. "We'll see what happens. I feel nervous. I am kind of scared. I hear good and bad stories. It just worries me. I don't tolerate pain well. I have to think of the long term."

In the holding or preoperating area, a registered nurse reviewed pre-surgery restrictions and the names of any medicine she had been taking. He gave her several pamphlets, on pain management, the importance of walking after surgery, hospital-acquired infections, and a hospital program for patients to connect with administrators and others about issues during their stay. He also gave Rojas-Gudino a stomach-relaxing medicine to reduce any nausea. "Our goal is to make this as easy as possible on you," he said. Next came the placement of an intravenous or IV line through which many of her medicines for the surgery, including anesthesia, would be administered. "Don't think about it," he told her. "Just breathe and take big breaths."

Carpenter, her surgeon, stopped by to say hello and mark the height, depth, and width of each breast with an indelible marker. "You will have blue marks for weeks," Carpenter warned. She told her that she likely will go home from the hospital with two surgical drains because her plastic surgeon, Dr. Ivan Turpin, "is a two-drain person; most plastic surgeons use four drains, two on each side." In earlier appointments, she assessed Rojas-Gudino for lymphedema, a chronic postsurgery pain problem, and concluded she was not at risk.

The anesthesiologist for the surgery, Dr. Eric Wellmeyer, arrived next to examine her mouth, heart, and lungs and to discuss anesthesia and pain management, which includes numbing medicine much like the ones dentists use and regional nerve blocks to reduce postoperative pain. Anesthesia is tailored to each person's age, weight, medical history, current history of medications, and past experience with anesthesia, Wellmeyer said. Then he gave her a consent form to sign that allowed the use of anesthesia.

Squeamish of needles, Rojas-Gudino was assured she wouldn't be poked a lot because most of her medicines would be administered intravenously. Wellmeyer gave her a relaxing medicine, Midazolam, like valium, given through an IV.

It is known as "happy juice," he said.

———— ◈ ————

Several attendants team wheel Rojas-Gudino down a hallway to an operating room. A team moved her from a gurney to an operating table, where she was prepped for surgery.

Safety precautions include a scrubbing of her breasts with an antiseptic solution; compression devices wrapped around each of her calves to deter a surgery-related problem, deep vein thrombosis; and monitors that track important heart, breathing, and brain measurements. To further deter bacteria, the room was bone cold, requiring some staff to wear hospital jackets, even hospital blankets wrapped around their shoulders.

"We gave her pain medicine, fentanyl, and a little bit of lidocaine followed by propofol, our standard induction agent for anesthesia," Wellmeyer said. He also administered two regional nerve blocks, as he had discussed earlier with Rojas-Gudino.

She needed a breathing tube, inserted with a device called a laryngoscope, which is standard for longer operations to keep the airway open and "help breathe for her since her muscles are relaxed during the operation," Wellmeyer explained, as he placed the device in her mouth to move and hold her tongue out of place. When Rojas-Gudino lost consciousness, he put an oxygen mask over her mouth.

Before actual surgery started at about 3 p.m., the team began what hospitals call a timeout to review the name of the procedure planned and the body parts it involves. Two large poster boards in the OR list other essential review items. Carpenter even initials each breast she operated on as well with the letters *SN* to indicate which breast is used for a sentinel lymph node biopsy to see if cancer has spread. The test is not needed if there is no cancer.

Carpenter operated from a tray of instruments marked "Radical Breast Tray" that holds rows of scissors of varied sizes, retractors that the team uses to hold back tissue, and blades and sharp instruments of various sorts. She alternated between using scissors for fine work in areas she doesn't want to traumatize and a hand-held, electrically charged tool that both cuts and or uses heat to sear tissue, particularly in the beginning of the operation.

Her job is to remove all breast tissue under the skin from the collarbone to the incision she will make, and from the side of the breast under the arm to the breastbone in the center of the chest.

Surgeons use different types of incisions, depending on whether a tumor is present and a doctor's preference. Carpenter prefers incisions along the crease or inframammary fold because they leave the least visible scars. It is more technically challenging to perform a mastectomy with such an incision because the surgeon has to remove tissue high up into the chest. Incisions around the nipple, another approach, give more access to the breast but leave more visible scarring.

Before she cut, she squirted a numbing medicine into the breast to reduce pain. "It's the same solution they use for liposuction," she said. She guides herself with the earlier markings she put on Rojas-Gudino's chest as her boundaries.

"The breast is more of a pentagon," she said. "It has five sides. I find the place where the breast tapers in under the collarbone. Sometimes the smaller breasted patients are harder to do because there's less space."

"What we have to do as surgeons is to think about the nipple as just another margin," said Carpenter, who has been doing nipple-sparing mastectomy for about seven years.

"If it's just another margin and if that tumor is not too close to it, we don't need to take the nipple. It's another potential operation to go back and remove the nipple. As long as they are comfortable going into the operation with their eyes open, knowing the potential to have a second operation exists, I'll do it."

Carpenter worked on one breast at a time. To remove tissue high up in the breast, she had to bend and crouch to see with the help of a high-powered headlight affixed to her surgical head gear. She also asked Wellmeyer to rotate the table to improve her vantage point. It took her two hours for the mastectomy portion of the surgery.

"I won the battle," she said, as she removed a breast tissue specimen. Carpenter gave it to a nurse who tagged it and placed it into a large plastic container for pathologists to review. All tissue is checked for cancer, just to be sure.

The second breast went a little more smoothly because Carpenter said she learned from the first side and made the incision in the second breast slightly wider.

Throughout the surgery, the team accounted for every tool, even the gauze sponges used in the surgery, as protection against leaving items inside a patient. The sponges have microchips implanted in them so that staff can pass a wand over a person "to be sure nothing's left behind," Wellmeyer said.

In final steps, Carpenter squirted the pocket she created with more numbing medicine.

"Usually I can tell on the first day after surgery if a nipple will live or die," she said. "If it looks like it wants to die, it gets more bruised-looking than the rest of the breast," she said. "You almost get a sense that it doesn't look like it's going to live. But what we also know is that sometimes they still perk up and they still live. If it looks a little dark, we just wait to declare itself. Sometimes, it takes a few weeks. Most of the time, in my experience, by the time I see a woman in my office the next week, I'll have a better sense of whether it's going to live."

Carpenter instructed the staff to call Turpin, the plastic surgeon, to tell him he could begin his part of the surgery by 5 p.m.

He began with another timeout to review the plan for surgery. Then he examined the pockets Carpenter left him for the reconstruction portion of the surgery. He washed the breast cavity again with a diluted antiseptic solution.

The operation, like many implant reconstructions with expanders, will use a product called acellular dermal matrix, or ADM, made from sterilized human or animal collagen. It adds support and improves contour around an implant. It has been found effective in preventing or minimizing common implant problems, such as capsular contracture, when scar tissue forms around an implant, and distortion, when an implant shifts, particularly during exercise.

Turpin prefers using implants to autologous tissue for uncomplicated breast reconstruction cases and usually uses smooth, round implants instead of a new generation of anatomical implants, also called cohesive or gummy bear implants. "They rotate. It's hard to keep them properly oriented and they lack projection. I've had a fair amount of patient dissatisfaction with them and I've had to change them to conventional implants."

Turpin sutured a sheet of ADM to the edge of the pectoralis major muscle in the chest. Then he placed an expander, a temporary, adjustable saline implant used in most reconstruction, under the ADM material and the pectoralis major muscle.

To fill the implant, Turpin used a small magnetic tool that locates a metal port in the expander. He inserted a thin needle into the device so a nurse could fill it with a saline solution. Over the next three months, depending on how everything goes and what size breasts Rojas-Gudino desires, Turpin will add more saline solution before swapping out the temporary devices for permanent implants.

Turpin favors filling the implant a little bit at the time of mastectomy but not too much so that women wake up to see a fuller breast. Once the implants were in place he laid down a tube, or drain, next to the expander. Patients wear the drains for about a week, but sometimes longer. The tubes are attached to drainage bulbs that collect fluid. It's 6:15 p.m., four hours and fifteen minutes after Rojas-Gudino was taken to the OR.

After stitching the mastectomy incision closed with small sutures, Turpin asked the staff to sit Rojas-Gudino up so he can see her breast symmetry. Satisfied, he asked staff to call Victor Gudino to meet him in a nearby conference room.

He walked Gudino through the answers to typical questions: "The nerve blocks she got will keep her pretty comfortable," he began. "She won't need any narcotics and hopefully will avoid getting an upset stomach."

Turpin told Gudino that Veronica "looked good. The tissues were healthy. We already pumped her up a little. There's nothing for you to do when she goes home except to empty the drain and the nurses will show you how to do that. I'll see her next week, usually on Thursday. At home, all she should do is sit around and relax. Tonight, she's not going to feel great and she'll want to sleep."

Doctors give patients different restrictions. Turpin does not like his patients to shower while their surgery drains are in, even if they cover them with a garbage bag, as some Internet sites recommend, or showering backward, with drains away from the faucet. He fears it risks infection. Sponge baths are preferred.

Otherwise, he does not set many limits. "I don't restrict them at all, if they are off narcotics," he told Gudino. "If they are comfortable, I let them drive. I'm pretty liberal. She will be sore so I don't really have to tell them to take it easy. Many patients feel good and I have to slow them down a little bit until we take the drains out. Drains are in seven to ten days usually. Maybe by next Thursday, I can get them out if they don't drain much. We didn't do any lymph node surgery today so she may not drain a lot."

"I won't add saline to her expanders again until about the third week. That's kind of my protocol. I like them feeling good. Some surgeons expand right away. That doesn't add anything. It is just more painful when it's done early. I have filled her tissue expanders quite a bit already. She won't need too much more saline added to her expanders."

"My biggest concern the first two weeks is the circulation to the nipple. Dr. Carpenter has to take out all the breast tissue under the nipple without cutting its blood supply. We watch that. Some may turn a little blue but they pink up. I don't think we will have any trouble here, but you may have to remove the nipple. She's healthy and shouldn't have a problem. Smokers, diabetics and larger breasted women present the most problems, especially if I have to move the nipple a long way to get it back up on the chest."

He concluded by telling Gudino, "She is a pretty straightforward case for a prophylactic nipple-sparing mastectomy with immediate reconstruction." Earlier, Carpenter had called the surgery "a textbook case" for a mastectomy.

Rojas-Gudino spent the night in the hospital and took it easy at home in her first week. The worst part were the surgical drains, she said. When her doctor took them out a week later, she felt immediate relief, and that night, she slept soundly without them. "It was a mental thing," she said. "I worried I was going to pull the drains out. I worried they'd get infected. They looked very strange. I didn't like them but I had no choice but keep them in."

Surgery left her with so little strength at first that "I did not have the strength to open the refrigerator door or the door on my car." A week later, she was moving a little better. "I can move my arms a little. It's a day at a time."

The first four days after surgery, she was in pain, particularly under her breast where her incisions were. She had difficulty moving around and using her arms, she said.

Three weeks later, she wrote in an email, "I still feel pain and I'm uncomfortable. The highest degree of pain was felt the first four days after surgery. The pain medicine helped, but I just hated the feeling of being drugged up. When I took Percocet, I felt drowsy and sleepy so after the fourth day I started taking extra-strength Tylenol. I still take it at night; it helps me sleep and tolerate the discomfort of laying down." At three weeks postop, her pain moved to her chest cavity, she said. "All the stitching inside must be healing up, plus trying to move and making my arm useful again which certainly produces pain. It does get better day by day but I'm not 100% pain-free yet."

Otherwise, she and her doctors are pleased with the results. "They said everything is wonderful," she said, after appointments with both doctors one week after surgery. "They said I'm going to be so satisfied with the end results. Everything is healing properly."

Turpin said he'd fill her expander with a little more saline water at her next appointment. But already, she could see she will get slightly larger breasts, which is OK with her. "Yes, I'm actually looking forward to that."

She was asked, "Are you ready to work it?"

"Yes," she said with a laugh. "I am."

MASTECTOMY RESOURCES

- What to expect: www.breastcancer.org; www.komen.org
- Discharge tips: http://www.nlm.nih.gov/medlineplus/ency/patientinstructions/000244.htm

4

A Veteran's Story: Lumpectomy

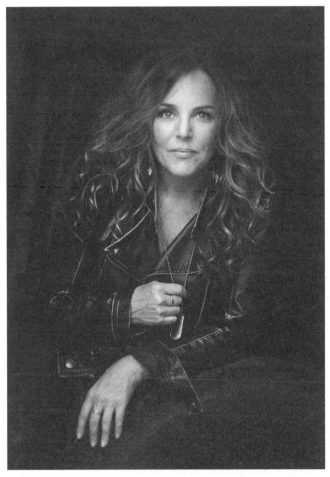

Kathleen Galligan is an army veteran who wonders if she got breast cancer from exposure to toxic substances on a U.S. military base. Photo by Erin Galligan.

BY KATHLEEN GALLIGAN

Author's note: The spotlight isn't my happy place. I'm very private. Or was. My modesty went out the window after months of treatment for breast cancer at Henry Ford West Bloomfield Hospital where most of the exceptional human beings in the oncology, surgery, and radiology departments wouldn't recognize me with a shirt on. I agreed to do this chapter in part under duress. I think there may have been wine or anesthesia involved. But my real motivation came when I discovered an unexpected risk factor I could not, in good conscience, be silent about. I also looked at the women in the other chapters and thought it an honor to be counted among them.

Call it the Luck of the Irish, Murphy's Law, whatever you like. The timing was ironic. Five months into photographing women for a book about breast cancer—Wouldn't you bloody know it?—I was diagnosed with the same damned thing.

There had been no signs of a problem. No symptoms. No lumps. Nothing. Cheryl Perkins, the gorgeous nurse from Detroit I photographed for chapter 1, made me promise to schedule a slightly overdue mammogram. It seemed routine.

And then the call. Breast cancer. Me. My family specializes in lung cancer, depression, and the national pastime of the Irish. We are not breast cancer people. Other people get that. And now I was part of that Other.

My odds of having breast cancer weren't as low as it seemed. The average American woman has a one in eight chance of getting it in her lifetime. But I'm also a veteran, a former army medic, and according to a 2009 study, doctors at Walter Reed Army Medical Center found that breast cancer rates among military women are 20 to 40 percent higher than their civilian counterparts.[1] And while more than 800 women were wounded in Iraq and Afghanistan from 2000 to 2011, 874 were diagnosed with breast cancer, according to the Armed Forces Health Surveillance Center. That blows my mind.[2]

Before I hung up my fatigues in 1987, I spent two-and-a-half years at Fort Devens. The base may not have the notoriety of Camp Lejeune, where breast cancer was found in eighty male marines. And it isn't Fort McClellan with thousands of sick veterans calling themselves "toxic soldiers." All the same, it contained a stew of carcinogens: arsenic, mercury, cadmium, toluene, and trichloroethylene. Poison circulated above and below the water table. It was added to the EPA's National Priorities List in 1989, and cleanup continues to this day. Lovely. I'd been living on a toxic Superfund site. Maybe the irony is that I didn't get cancer sooner. I'm proud that I served. My dog tags are dearer to me than any piece of jewelry could ever be. But I'm angry that the U.S. Department of Defense, one of the world's greatest polluters, poisons its own. If you are one of us, keep up on yearly exams.

Napoleon once said, "A soldier will fight long and hard for a bit of colored ribbon." No one expected that ribbon to be pink.

I never was the pink type. My friend Stella, who's covered conflict from Chechnya to Mogadishu, said, "If I were cancer I wouldn't want to meet you in a dark alley." It was a vote of confidence I needed. The possibility of a mastectomy didn't scare me. I just wanted to get rid of cancer—the faster the better. My surgeon was a wonderful man, Dr. Robert Elkus, who wore running shoes everyday while he worked from dawn until dusk and spoke to me like I was family. He advised against mastectomy because survival rates were no better in my case and lumpectomy involved far less surgery and trauma. My decision came down to test results, the advice of a surgeon I trust, and damned good luck.

Following that advice, a few days later I was prepping for surgery. A lot of people compare cancer to a roller coaster ride. It's more like a joy ride with a drunken driver. Mine started early on a Wednesday, and I was less than enthusiastic about the switch from producing the book to being featured in it. I felt less anxious about the actual surgery that morning than the entourage of family and bystanders around me. I'd agreed to allow my surgery to become part of the book. I was delighted to meet the anesthesiologist. When I woke, the cancerous tissue and three lymph nodes had already been sent to the lab. Then I waited for test results. There was a lot of waiting involved. Dr. Elkus was kind enough to call late that Friday evening so my weekend wasn't spent worrying about my top concern. "I have some good news," he said. The lymph nodes were clear. The cancer hadn't spread, and I was riding a high.

As the other tests came back, I learned that I had estrogen-positive early-stage invasive ductal carcinoma. It's really not as impressive as it sounds. As cancer goes, it's pretty uninspired, but I'd need a second surgery to catch the rebellious cells that eluded us. Dr. Elkus took that bit of news much harder than I did. I was given a few weeks to heal before the next surgery—just in time for cancer awareness month. Believe me when I say I was aware. While other people enjoyed the fall colors last year, I saw nothing but pink.

They put me on the estrogen blocker Tamoxifen to prevent recurrence, and I went back to work. The week I began taking it, I was staked out in front of the federal courthouse in downtown Detroit with other news media. I hadn't been there since I covered a prominent oncologist who was convicted of poisoning his patients for money. As we say in the business, you can't make this shit up. A wave of nausea hit, and I scanned a nearby parking lot for a semiprivate trash can to hurl in. For weeks it continued.

I dreaded the possibility of chemo. Burn me, cut me. But please keep the poison away. At one time they blasted everyone with it. Now there's a test, called oncotyping, that gives a recurrence score between 1 and 100. If the score is low, the benefits don't outweigh the side effects. I was shooting for a big fat zero. A bit of my cancer was shipped to a lab for an eternity of waiting on that number to come in. Life stands still for lab results, and sister, the lab ain't open on the weekend. I tried to resign myself to the possibility of chemo and losing my hair, my eyebrows, and eyelashes. That seemed worse than mastectomy somehow. I could handle being sick. I hated the thought of looking the part. I bought a Conehead wig figuring if it had to happen, I might as well go big.

Fortunately, my odds of recurrence turned out to be very low. I was spared from chemo, mastectomy, and reconstruction. A couple of surgeries and a season of radiation—that's like winning the cancer lottery.

Although the second surgery went well, Tamoxifen made me feel like holy hell. The nausea was somewhat manageable, but I was beginning to get very depressed. Something wasn't right. I decided to laugh about my situation to keep from losing my mind. My coworkers at the *Detroit Free Press* had organized a campaign to bring meals to my home after I returned from both surgeries. I loved their visits. My little house was filled with life. "Hell," I joked, "had I known it would be this much fun, I'd have done it years ago." Friends I hadn't heard from in years reached out to me. People brought candy, books, movies, candles, and wine. It was overwhelming. At one point, there were so many flowers I ran out of vases and bottles and mason jars. I was often moved to tears by their kindness. I still am, and I will never forget it.

Maybe it's the soldier in me, but I'm not in the habit of reaching out for help so all the unsolicited spoiling was wonderful. Denial works for me. Although I made sure to get the best care I could, for the most part I lived like the cancer didn't exist. I was actually doing things for other people because I was "OK." I started to repaint rooms at my (then) boyfriend's house. And I got busy fund-raising for this book as I watched the leaves pile up, the snow pile up, and the bills pile up.

From the time I was diagnosed, cancer felt like a twisted publicity stunt for this book. I promise it wasn't. I had just enough cancer cred to be legit, but compared to what other women experience, it felt like cheating. I referred to it as "my candy-ass cancer." I fooled myself into thinking I was invincible. I'm a veteran dammit. I'm a photojournalist. I'm a strong woman.

Bullshit.

I'm human.

Friends said, "If you need anything, I'm here." Did I ask for help? Hell no. I'm a trooper. And a fool. I raked leaves and shoveled snow between coats of paint, and I continued the march right through a ministroke somewhere between surgery two and surgery three. Just before Christmas while talking to a friend, my words became garbled midsentence. My whole right side went limp for about five minutes. They called it a TIA or "ministroke." I called it the worst five minutes of the past year. It was terrifying. It was the drug. They took me off of it immediately.

But my breed of breast cancer is estrogen positive. In other words, it feeds on estrogen. Loves the hell out of it. Estrogen was an enemy, and mine had to go. Without Tamoxifen to block it, we scheduled another surgery to remove my ovaries. I didn't realize how much I liked my estrogen. I miss it so.

Good-bye, ovaries. So long, estrogen. Hello, instant menopause on steroids.

Still, menopause was not going to affect me in the slightest. Not this girl. No sir, not me. My grandma once told me the seventeen-year-old in you never dies. It stuck. I'm a fifty-one-year-old grandma now, but menopause was completely out of sync with my happy teenage delusions.

Before this menopause business I slept like a baby. Now a typical night is interrupted with a dozen hot flashes. No sooner do I get back to sleep than I'm shivering on damp sheets wide awake with a pile of blankets kicked to the floor. Rinse. Wash. Repeat. I feel dehydrated. I walk around in a loopy fog.

Memory and focus left with my hormones and ability to sleep. I get dumber by the day, I swear. I don't recall the name of the person I met two seconds ago. I can't remember where I left my keys. My coworkers tease me about my little white desk fan, but I'm telling you, it's my new best friend. I'm glad they're amused. I may have escaped chemo brain; I'm afraid, however, that I've lost my mind to menopause.

Radiation? A breeze for me. I absolutely loved the radiation team and was in awe of the technology. In keeping with the denial theme, radiation involves invisible subatomic particles. I never saw what hit me. On the first round, I took my place on the linear accelerator table like some half-naked astronaut and waited for the laser show. The radiation therapist didn't get my reference to the film *2001: A Space Odyssey*. (Am I really that old?) But when he went into the control room, he found the theme song on his iPhone and played it over the sound system. I looked up to see a calming photo of a wooded country road. The staff hid a Where's Waldo figure among the trees in it and moved him around from week to week for our entertainment. They took away any fear. I joked with them that they actually made cancer fun. I miss my Tuesday talks with my favorite doctor, Dr. Levin. And I have to add that the parking was fabulous and the radiation side effects were nothing worse than sunburn and a few small blisters. The unexpected fatigue, on the other hand, absolutely hammered me. I still feel it six months later.

During the fall, winter, and spring I was focused on the mission. Time stood still. I went from one appointment or treatment to the next, and there were always more tests. I couldn't wait to get my life back and feel like me again. I put on makeup and a smile to give the illusion of having my act together. You'd think I'd smarten up and admit I needed reinforcements once in a while. My brother tried. He wanted me to come stay with him from the beginning. He doesn't say things like, "I love you," but he was by my side for every surgery. Rather than ask if I wanted his help, he said he'd be doing the driving. I love him for that.

Then it all just stopped. The fight was over. No more surgery or radiation or miserable medications. I went back to real time, and I found myself alone wondering, "Now what?"

Maybe it's natural to expect to just pick up where you left off before cancer invades your breast and your life. But the transition is unfamiliar territory. Other survivors have told me the same thing. We will never be the same. There's all this talk about a "new normal" after cancer. I'm not there yet.

I decided to make a few changes to my old normal. During a road trip for this book, my friend Michelle, her fiancé, Balam, and I had just pulled into a drugstore to get water and stretch. My son Zack called. He wanted to know if I was mad at him because I hadn't visited him or my granddaughters in a while. I lost it. I was doing such a good job of downplaying cancer that he thought I was avoiding him. He took it personally. The truth is, I was exhausted and didn't want either my family or friends to see it or waste energy worrying. I bit my lip as I fought back tears. By the time I hung up, they were running down my face.

Michelle saw the tears. When she came back to the car she had three red clown noses in the bag. We took a ridiculous photo with the noses and uploaded it to Facebook. Within minutes, Marjorie Hacker, who we had photographed for chapter 8, saw it, photoshopped herself into the shot, and reposted it. I love these women.

I finally got it through my thick skull that I was hurting people I loved most by putting up a false front of strength. I missed my family, and I needed to be with them. I was missing the best parts of my own life. It's not strength to go it alone. Vulnerability takes courage. This is no revelation to any well-adjusted person, but I've been epically gutless about it. We all have our own forms of crazy—this is one of mine. I'm still not great at saying, "Hey, I could use a hand here," but I'm at least to the point where I can say, "Give me a break just for now. This is scary shit and I feel lost."

Cancer's been good to me. It was a swift kick in the ass gift-wrapped in a few mutant cells. The crazy thing is I'm happier than ever. I'm aware of how fortunate I am. My lazy, unambitious cancer was caught before it gained momentum. I'm alive. I don't mind the changes, and I don't mind the scar tissue that feels like a rock in my boob. I'm grateful I still have two. Perfection is overrated. I'm more comfortable in my skin now than I've ever been. Maybe I just appreciate how much of it I still have.

I've heard scars are tattoos with a better story. Is it possible I even feel affection for my scars? It is. I love them. My scars are a permanent reminder of my latest adventure, a time where I felt more love than ever before. They connect me to millions of others who share the experience. My scars give me permission to be vulnerable. They remind me of the countless times people went out of their way to show me kindness. They don't make me feel less of a woman. They make me feel more of a human being. I've got people. There's no medal or ribbon for any of them, but I cherish every last cut, burn, and dent. They are my proof. I'm one of the lucky ones.

And I'm still standin'.

5

Reconstruction with Tissue

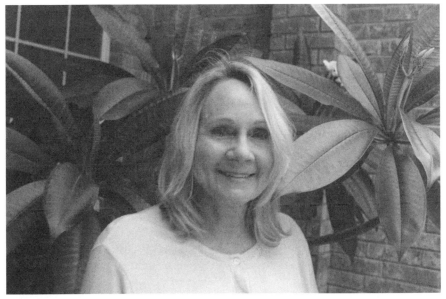

Kim Land didn't want a nipple-sparing mastectomy, worrying it could leave cancer behind. Photo supplied by Kim Land.

Five weeks after her mother died of breast cancer, Kim Land felt "something's wrong with my left breast." She wondered if she was just imagining it because she had a clean mammogram three months earlier.

Land, fifty-five, of San Antonio, a certified public accountant, waited three months.

When she couldn't shake the feeling something was wrong, she made an appointment with her doctor just to be sure.

An exam found nothing, but "just to pacify me," her doctor prescribed a more definitive, three-dimensional mammogram, which found a suspicious area. A biopsy confirmed it was a small tumor. She had a choice of lumpectomy, but she didn't want radiation, having seen her father live with radiation damage to his chest years ago, she said.

For Land and a group of highly motivated breast cancer patients, the best choice was mastectomy and breast reconstruction using her own abdominal tissue. She also decided to have a prophylactic mastectomy on the other side. She underwent bilateral skin-sparing mastectomies and immediate reconstruction with SIEA flaps, one of the newer, more complicated, tissue-based reconstruction techniques, using the superficial inferior epigastric blood vessels in her lower abdomen and the lower abdominal tissue, like the tissue removed in a tummy tuck.

Land had the procedure June 31, 2015, at Methodist Hospital, San Antonio, the operating home for PRMA Plastic Surgery, one of the leading breast reconstruction practices in the world.

WHAT IS MICROSURGERY?

Microsurgery is a subspecialty within plastic surgery that allows doctors to transplant tissue and surrounding blood vessels from one part of the body to another. The surgery is done with high-powered magnification microscopes and high-magnification operating eyeglasses known as "loupes," special instruments, sutures, or surgical thread finer than a human hair, and operating room TV screens that carry live images of the surgery.

Not all plastic surgeons perform microsurgery, and ones that do may not offer all tissue-based breast reconstruction procedures. To find a microvascular surgeon, go to http://www.microsurg.org, the website of the American Society for Reconstructive Microsurgery.

Reconstruction using her own tissue "seemed like the right thing for me," said Land, a mother of two grown children, a cyclist, and runner who participates in half-marathons and two-day fitness events. Implant reconstruction didn't appeal to her. A sister's breast implants shifted sideways during a Colorado ski trip, she said, explaining her choice.

Tissue-based reconstruction is by far the less popular reconstruction choice in the United States. Only 19,066 of the 102,215 reconstruction procedures performed in 2014 in the United States were tissue based, according to the American Society of Plastic Surgeons (ASPS).[1] The rest had implant reconstruction out of choice or lack of access to other options.

Autologous procedures, as they are also called, use a person's own tissue to make one or two new breasts. This tissue, known in plastic surgery as flaps, may be taken from the lower abdomen, inner or back of the thigh, butt, or back.

TISSUE RECONSTRUCTION METHODS

Lower abdominal tissue has been used for breast reconstruction for several decades. The earliest was the "TRAM" flap, a procedure that sacrifices one or both abdominal (*Transverse Rectus Abdominis Myocutaneous*) muscles. The TRAM flap is performed today in one of three forms: pedicled TRAM, free TRAM, and muscle-sparing free TRAM. The main differences between these three procedures are the amount of abdominal muscle removed and how the tissue is transferred to the chest. Studies have shown that the degree of loss in abdominal strength following TRAM surgery mirrors the amount of abdominal muscle removed. In 2014, 4,939 TRAM flap procedures were performed in the United States, the third most common type of flap procedure, after DIEP and back (latissimus) flaps, according to data from the American Society of Plastic Surgeons (ASPS).

The DIEP flap, and the less invasive SIEA flap, transfer lower abdominal skin and fat but, unlike the TRAM flap, preserve all the abdominal muscle. They involve disconnecting the "flap" of tissue from the body, transplanting it to the chest, and reconnecting the blood vessels using microsurgery. The DIEP flap gets its blood supply from the *Deep Inferior Epigastric Perforator* blood vessels in the abdomen. Plastic surgeons at leading centers say the DIEP is the preferred method of tissue-based reconstruction widely performed by most plastic surgeons.

Recovery from a tissue-based procedure takes about six weeks before women return to near-normal functions. It is a challenge that some women, particularly younger, motivated, and more educated ones, say they are up for, and are even willing to travel and possibly pay more for.

"Women often self-select for the procedure," said Dr. Minas Chrysopoulo, Land's microvascular plastic surgeon with PRMA Plastic Surgery in San Antonio. PRMA performs over six hundred microsurgical flap breast reconstructions a year. Some 550 of these procedures are DIEP flaps.

Many women reject tissue-based reconstruction, primarily because abdominal methods leave a hip-to-hip scar, even when done by the best plastic surgeons.

Ideally, an abdominal incision from tissue-based reconstruction is several inches below the belly button just above the pubic hairline where it's less visible, extending across the abdomen from side to side. Making a lower scar is more technically challenging in women who don't have ideal tissue distribution, so they may be left with scars slightly higher in the abdomen, doctors say.

Regardless, "a scar is always going to be there," Chrysopoulo said. "In some women, it's almost imperceptible. Older women with fair skin tend to heal the best. Younger women or dark-skinned women tend to have an increased risk of more visible scarring or pigmentation changes. Many women don't care. They are looking at what they consider to be the bigger picture. But for other women it's a deal-breaker. I have found that the best way to communicate the possible appearance and location of the final scar is to show pictures of previous patients."

Women who want flap-based procedures often are equally adamant about why they would never want silicone implants, rejecting them as foreign.

"It's very common in my practice, at the beginning of the consultation for patients to tell me, off the bat, implants aren't an option," Chrysopoulo said. "That's one reconstructive option that is immediately out for them. It's very clear they want to use their own tissue for very specific reasons, usually to obtain the most natural results."

Women attracted to tissue-based reconstruction like it because it "gives a life-long reconstruction," said Dr. Joseph Disa, a microvascular plastic surgeon at Memorial Sloan Kettering Cancer Center, New York.

"It's living tissue. It's soft. It's warm. It will change in size and volume with the patient. If a patient gains weight, the flaps get a little bigger. If a patient loses weight, it gets a little smaller. It's normal tissue. I also tell patients that based on my experience and what's reported in the literature, patient satisfaction with their breast reconstruction over time, if they had a flap reconstruction it goes up over time whereas if they had implants, it goes down over time."

When presenting reconstruction options, Dr. Adeyiza Momoh, a microvascular plastic surgeon at the University of Michigan in Ann Arbor, tells women to consider the time they will spend recovering from a flap procedure with time they will save later visiting their plastic surgeon for implant-related issues over the years.

"When I talk to patients, I tell them, 'you are going to be investing time and effort into this,'" he said. "You either invest that time and effort up front and do the reconstruction now or you invest less time now but more later. With implant-based reconstruction, you recover faster. It's simpler. But ultimately, long term, we see these patients over and over again for maintenance issues. The implants rupture.

There's the issue of capsular contracture" or hardening of scar tissue around the implant. "Those are the two big complications that need additional operations in the future. Autologous reconstruction is a longer operation and recovery but once you are done, it's a very rare situation where we will see you 10 or 15 years down the line for revisions."

＝＝◆＝＝

There are a half-dozen ways to make a breast with a woman's own tissue from her abdomen, thighs, back, or butt.

Here are the names of autologous tissue procedures and a brief description:

Abdominal techniques:

- TRAM flap, or transverse rectus abdominis myocutaneous flap. There are three types:
  - Pedicled TRAM flap: One of the early types of tissue-based reconstruction, the pedicled TRAM flap takes skin, fat, the abdominal muscle and overlying fascia and tunnels it under the upper abdominal skin to the chest. No microsurgery is involved.
  - Free TRAM flap: This procedure uses the same tissue as the pedicled TRAM but instead of tunneling the flap to the chest, the flap is disconnected from the patient's body, transplanted to the chest, and reconnected using microsurgery. The main advantage over the pedicled TRAM is improved blood supply. Since there is no tunneling under the skin as there is with the pedicled procedure, there is no subsequent upper abdominal bulge around the rib cage area, which is often seen with tunneling.
  - Muscle-sparing free TRAM flap: A similar procedure to the free TRAM that takes a smaller portion of the muscle, with or without the overlying fascia. The advantage over the free TRAM is that this procedure preserves some of the abdominal muscle. The tissue is removed from its blood supply and brought up to the breast pocket, where blood flow is restored by reconnecting the artery and vein.
- DIEP, or deep inferior epigastric perforator flap. This uses the same lower abdominal skin and fat as a TRAM flap, but unlike the TRAM, preserves *all* of the underlying abdominal

muscle(s). The flap and its blood supply (deep inferior epigastric artery and vein) are disconnected from the abdomen, transplanted to the chest, and reconnected to the blood vessels in the chest using microsurgery.

- SIEA, or superficial inferior epigastric artery flap. This flap is similar to the DIEP flap except for the blood supply. The SIEA blood vessels are found in the fatty tissue between skin and the abdominal fascia, compared to the DIEP blood vessels that run below and within the abdominal muscle. While the surgical preparation is slightly different, both procedures spare the abdominal muscles and only use the patient's skin and fat to reconstruct a breast.

Other flap techniques:

- Buttocks. IGAP/SGAP: Inferior gluteal artery perforator (IGAP) flap and the superior gluteal artery perforator (SGAP) flap. These are flaps of skin, fat, and associated blood vessels taken from the buttocks. Depending on where you have the most excess tissue, the flaps can be taken from either the upper portion of the buttock, which is supplied by the blood vessels known as the superior gluteal artery and vein, or from the lower portion of the buttock, which is supplied by the inferior gluteal artery flap.
- Back. The latissimus dorsi procedure takes skin, fat, and muscle below the shoulder blade known as the latissimus dorsi muscle, and tunnels it through the armpit to the chest, with the arteries and veins attached. The location of the incision on the back will depend on the amount of skin that is needed to replace the skin removed during the mastectomy. No microsurgery is involved.
- Thigh. A TUG or transverse upper gracilis flap uses tissue from the inner portion of the upper thigh and typically is offered to women who aren't candidates for DIEP or SIEA flaps. A related procedure is the PAP flap, or profunda artery perforator flap, that uses tissue from the back of the upper thigh, beneath the buttock crease. It is a new procedure gaining in popularity, particularly in thinner patients who are not good candidates for DIEP flap reconstruction.

The field has brought some of the biggest changes in breast construction in years, as significant as the development of silicone implants in the 1960s. It builds on fifty years of microsurgery advances in which plastic surgeons developed new ways to repair damaged ears, cheekbones, eyes, and other body features with swathes of tissue and connecting blood vessels taken from elsewhere in the body.

"I can make a breast from almost anything," said Dr. Kongrit Chaiyasate, a microvascular plastic surgeon with the Beaumont Health system in Royal Oak, Michigan, who borrows techniques he uses in complex facial reconstruction to make new breasts. While he has gained notoriety for his facial reconstruction cases, including a girl whose face was badly mauled by a raccoon, more than 80 percent of his business is breast reconstruction, mostly tissue based. He wishes more women heard about the option from their breast surgeons. "Women aren't told about all their options," he said. "When a woman is sent to me, I discuss all the options. There are pros and cons. Reconstruction with implants is quicker, women get back to the baseline faster but unfortunately there's a large revision rate in 10 years. It's the hardware. It's subject to rupture and other complications. It's a foreign body."

Twenty years ago, autologous breast reconstruction was a long operation with a long, arduous recovery, because it usually involved removing a flap of tissue with the entire muscle or part of it and its blood supply.

In 2014, there were 7,866 breast reconstructions performed with DIEP flaps, compared to 5,572 back or latissimus dorsi flap operations; 4,939 TRAM flap operations that sacrifice one or both abdominal Transverse Rectus Abdominis Myocutaneous muscles in the abdomen, and 689 "other" procedures, according to the ASPS database. In contrast, 83,149 reconstructions were performed with breast implants.

Because of complications, particularly hernias and loss of abdominal strength, of TRAM flap operations, top teams and centers no longer perform TRAM procedures, including those in San Antonio and at St. Charles Surgical Hospital in New Orleans, another high-volume breast reconstruction center.

"There's no question implants can give you a very good reconstruction," said Chrysopoulo, Land's plastic surgeon.

"For the right person, it can be a great option and patients can get a really nice result. But, generally speaking, implants have issues that tissue reconstruction doesn't. Many implants get hard over time, causing deformity and even pain. Breasts reconstructed with implants can feel cold, visible implant rippling is common, and the implants can rupture. The implant companies recommend that they be removed and replaced every 10 years."

"By comparison, tissue doesn't get ripples. It won't rupture. It doesn't feel cold. It increases and decreases in size with weight change. It ages with you. Some people would argue the DIEP flap is the gold standard period, not just for tissue reconstruction."

Weight, body mass index, amount or distribution of body fat, and other factors may rule out women for tissue options. Many centers use a BMI cutoff of 30 for eligibility standards, Chrysopoulo said.

PRMA uses a BMI of 40 as a cutoff, Chrysopoulo said. "A high BMI does increase your risk of complications with any surgery, and breast reconstruction is no different. I'm not saying it's risk-free. You have to have an in-depth conversation with the patient so they understand that because of their weight, there is a higher co-morbidity overall. Higher BMI patients have a higher risk of problems like wound healing."

Research published by the group in 2012 found no difference in flap complications among heavier women.[2] "Higher BMI, in our practice, doesn't increase flap-related complications," Chrysopoulo said. "Our flap success, abdominal bulge and abdominal hernia rates are the same across the BMI spectrum. As long as patients are educated about their risks, they can be DIEP flap candidates up to a BMI of 40."

Thin women, by comparison, may not have enough abdominal tissue or the right abdominal tissue distribution to reconstruct one or both breasts, he said. "It depends on your expectations and goals," Chrysopoulo said. "If your BMI is less than 20, you don't have much tissue over your lower abdomen, you have D-cup breasts and it's important for you to maintain that size, you won't be a good candidate. You'll need a combination of flaps, or flaps and fat grafting."

In New York, Disa, uses a variety of measurements, including what he called a "pinch test" of belly fat to determine eligibility for a DIEP flap.

"It's not simply based on weight or body mass index," he said. "It depends on where the patient's extra tissue is. If they have a little extra fat in their lower abdomen, and when you do what we call the pinch test, in the area below your umbilicus, you can create a ratio of that to the size of a patient's breast. You make a decision about whether it's a doable thing or not. Some patients have enough tissue to make a breast that's bigger than what they already have because they have small breasts but a lot of tissue in their abdomen."

Heavier women have higher rates of problems with pedicled TRAM flaps, including flap necrosis, in which the tissue that is transferred fails, typically because of poor blood supply, and the flap must be removed or enhanced with another flap, Disa said.

⸻ ◉ ⸻

Land's gynecologist referred her to Dr. Joe Johnston, a breast surgeon who works almost exclusively with Chrysopoulo for breast reconstruction cases. "I didn't shop around," said Land, who has two grown children. "I think I found them through the grace of God."

She met with Chrysopoulo and Johnston and liked them immediately, she said. In the presurgery appointments and on the morning of surgery, Land laid out her thoughts:

- She didn't want implants.
- She wouldn't mind increasing her bust size from a B to a C. Chrysopoulo said that it was likely he could make her a little bigger, as she requested. Like nearly all others, she will return in three months for her stage two reconstruction, or "fine-tuning," including fat-grafting techniques to improve shape, symmetry, and cosmetic appearance.
- She didn't want nipple-sparing mastectomies. "If I am going to go the route of having mastectomies, why would I keep something that possibly could still someday cause cancer? It just didn't feel right. I've never been that crazy about my nipples to start with."
- She was leaning toward tattoos, not conventional nipple reconstruction. "I've seen some lotus-type flowers that I think are phenomenally beautiful. It rang a bell with me because I'm not going to be the same. I don't want to pretend by putting in the nipple and areola I didn't have cancer." She also said she always was "uncomfortable with nipples staring out. To me, it's very personal. I'm the one that's going to see them. I have several months before I get to that step. I'm 99.9% sure that's the route I'm going to take."

Land said she and her husband prepared for the surgery in the weeks leading up to it. "We bought a shower chair. I've read all the manuals and everything I can to prepare, to know what to expect. I think that's the hardest part. I found most of what I needed on Dr. C's website," she said, referring to Chrysopoulo by the name many of his patients use for him.

Johnston finished the pre-op talk with Land by telling her and her husband that she won't be able to drive for two weeks and it will take two or three weeks to get back to her normal energy levels.

Land's surgery began just before 10 a.m., and ended by 4 p.m. The procedure is performed with general anesthesia and requires the placement of a breathing tube in the throat to maintain good breathing throughout a long operation. Patients also get IV sedatives, pain medicine, and a muscle relaxant.

Small sensor devices that stuck on her forehead like bandages measured the effectiveness of medicines to keep her unconscious. Each calf was wrapped with a compression device to deter a blood-clotting problem known as deep vein thrombosis.

At 9:55 a.m., Johnston began by making an incision around Land's nipple and areola and extended it down in a straight vertical line, almost to the crease, or inframammary fold, under her breast. Plastic surgeons debate and routinely revisit the question of the best way to make breast incisions, either in the inframammary fold, around the nipple and areola, extending from the nipple-areola, or some combination.

One of the most common is known as a lollipop incision. It works well for women getting a subsequent breast lift, Chrysopoulo said. Johnston confers with Chrysopoulo about each incision.

"I often include a breast lift as part of the second stage of breast reconstruction," Chrysopoulo said. "When we're planning a lift at stage 2 as we're planning for Mrs. Land's reconstruction, we place the initial mastectomy incision where the lollipop incision will be. This ensures scarring on the breast is kept to an absolute minimum."

Johnston worked quickly but effectively with staff that assists him in nearly all of his mastectomy procedures. "In doing a mastectomy, the most important part of making that pocket is recognizing those planes between the subcutaneous fat and breast tissue," Johnston said. "The second part is having the communication with your reconstructive surgeon."

Once her breast tissue had been removed, Johnston worked to get a small number of Land's lymph nodes, so-called sentinel lymph nodes, buried deep in the axilla or armpit. The lymph nodes are sent to pathology to determine if the tumor has spread beyond the breast.

The initial pathology results from this specimen, known as frozen section, are about 95 percent accurate and were delivered to the operating room within a few minutes.

The results brought great news for Land: no cancer in her sentinel lymph nodes.

Sentinel lymph node biopsy, now the standard of care, removes a very small number of lymph nodes, compared to a dozen or more a decade or more ago, a procedure that often led to chronic pain and swollen arm and chest problems.

It will take a few days before the final pathology results from the surgery are confirmed, which will tell whether Land needs chemotherapy.

Johnston gave a registered nurse two lymph nodes and two larger breast specimens, the main breast tissue he removed. Each specimen was placed in a separate plastic container and was marked to indicate the orientation of the tissue where it was obtained within the breast.

The mastectomy portion of the surgery went smoothly, with no hitches. Johnston finished the mastectomy in one hour, an operation that elsewhere might take 90 to 120 minutes.

He said there were no obvious signs of cancer from a tumor that he described as located in an eleven o'clock position of Land's upper breast quadrant. Cancer is not always apparent to the eye, he said. "There are subtleties in the way tissue behaves. It's the body's equivalent to inflammation. But I didn't notice anything there."

Before Johnston left the operating room, he placed a tissue specimen he removed from Land's chest on top of a flap of tissue Chrysopoulo marked on Land's abdomen.

It easily fit with the flap outlined in marking pen on Land's abdomen. The flap tissue was slightly larger to allow for a reconstructed breast that would be one cup size bigger than Land's original breasts, as she requested.

Like tag-team wrestlers, Chrysopoulo stepped forward. It was his turn to complete the next critical portion of the reconstruction—obtaining the flap by carefully dissecting the tissue in the abdomen, and then reconnecting the blood vessels in the flap to those in Land's chest.

First, he checked for any extra tiny pieces of breast tissue that might have been left. For safety's sake, he removed one tiny piece of breast tissue and gave it to be marked up as an additional pathology specimen.

Then, he returned to carefully dissecting the tissue in Land's abdomen. He operated with instruments powered by a foot pedal system that controls cutting and cauterizing tools, which he alternated using. He also used an instrument that releases small titanium clips he placed on blood vessels to keep them from bleeding.

Chrysopoulo pointed out the critical anatomy: the fascia, a tougher layer under the skin and fat, and just underneath that, the main muscle in the abdomen, the rectus abdominis muscle. It stretches from the top of the abdomen to the pubic bone in distinct groups—six distinct ones and possibly two more, hence the name *six-pack abs* sometimes used to describe these muscles.

Two main blood vessels provide blood to the lower abdominal tissue. The one most used in microsurgical abdominal flap breast reconstruction is the deep inferior epigastric artery and vein, which connect to smaller blood vessels known as perforators that travel through the rectus abdominis muscle to supply blood to the fatty layer and skin in the lower abdomen, Chrysopoulo explained.

The other blood vessel, the superficial inferior epigastric artery (SIEA), "runs much more superficially above the fascia and does not require doctors to dissect deeper into the abdominal muscle," Chrysopoulo said.

The more Chrysopoulo teased out the superficial blood vessels, the more he could see that Land would be fortunate enough to be a candidate for the less-invasive SIEA flap surgery.

About one in five women has SIEA vessels. Even fewer have vessels good enough to allow for the SIEA flap procedure, Chrysopoulo said. The SIEA flap has gained a foothold at top centers but can be very technically challenging to perform successfully and is not widely offered.

It was Land's lucky break. She had favorable SIEA anatomy on both sides. Avoiding an incision deeper into the abdomen "makes recovery even easier and eliminates any risk of bulging or hernia," Chrysopoulo said.

"The SIEA flap is based on superficial vessels. Instead of having to go down and dissect out the artery and vein within the muscle, this dissection remains above the abdominal wall fascia. She won't have the deeper incision, so her recovery should be even easier than after a DIEP flap," he said.

Once the tissue flaps were ready to be transferred, Chrysopoulo connected the SIEA flap blood vessels to the internal mammary arteries and veins in Land's chest.

He completed surgery by 4 p.m., pleased with the results and happy for Land that she was a bilateral SIEA flap candidate.

Most patients stay in the hospital for four days, he said. They get pain medicines but are encouraged early on to walk hospital floors. "Once she's near to going home, she'll be eating normally, showering. We tell our patients not to drive for two weeks. We have a six-week restriction on lifting. It's usually two-to-three weeks before energy levels start to come back. We have some women going back to work at four weeks and others at six weeks, depending on the physical requirements at work."

One in five of the San Antonio group's patients come from other regions of Texas or other states. The center helps out-of-towners with travel arrangements and discounts at local hotels, which it lists on its website, http://prma-enhance.com.

"It takes a lot for people to travel," Chrysopoulo said. "You have to be sure you have the right set-up for people to make it as safe as possible and to ensure the best outcomes. We may be in Texas but we're not cowboys when it comes to patient safety. We refused to jump into treating out-of-town patients until we had the right set up. Now a large number of the patients we treat come from out-of-town."

PRMA currently has arrangements with most of the larger insurers to be part of their physician referral networks, Chrysopoulo said. "We also have a strong interest in clinical research. We follow our patients extensively to create evidence-based standards for surgery aimed at constantly optimizing patient safety and outcomes."

Chrysopoulo said that of 5,722 DIEP flap procedures the team has performed since 1995, complications included:

- flap loss: less than 1 percent
- abdominal bulge: 0.2 percent

- abdominal hernia: 1.4 percent
- flap fat necrosis: 10 percent

Land found the first two days after her surgery a bit overwhelming managing and measuring fluid discharge from her surgical drains. She said she was happy to have an adjustable bed at home that made it easier to sleep in a somewhat upright position and get in and out of bed with less difficulty. "Simple tasks were exhausting. My first at-home shower was an ordeal. I was very glad that I had purchased a shower stool as by the time I undressed and managed the drains, with my sister's help, I was pretty much exhausted and needed to sit down. . . . but man did it feel wonderful! Afterwards, I absolutely had to rest for a couple of hours. It seemed like I would do a simple thing and then rest, do another simple thing and then rest."

A week after her surgery, Land said she was happy with the results. She planned to return to Chrysopoulo in three months for "some reshaping and so he can plump them up a bit," she said. Chrysopoulo told her that at her second stage of breast reconstruction he would lift her breasts and perform fat grafting, a procedure that liposuctions fat from another part of the body and reinjects it into the breasts to address contour defects, increase breast size, and improve the overall cosmetic results.

6

Medical Destinations

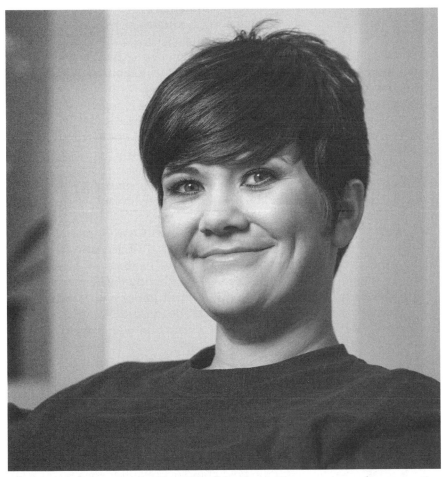

Katrina Bourn, her mother, and her sister all had breast cancer surgery and reconstruction at St. Charles Surgical Hospital, the world's only facility dedicated solely to breast cancer surgery and reconstruction. Photo supplied by St. Charles Surgical Hospital.

Ten years after Hurricane Katrina, Katrina Bourn, thirty-five, came to St. Charles Surgical Hospital in New Orleans for a preventive nipple-sparing bilateral mastectomy and reconstruction.

Her new breasts came from two sections of abdominal tissue, fat she didn't want anyway.

Bourn, a medical biller and mother of boys eleven and five, from Lena, Louisiana, in northern Louisiana, had waited since 2011 for this day.

That year, she learned she carries the BRCA1 mutation that significantly raises her risk of breast and ovarian cancer. She has an extensive family history of both tumors. Her grandmother survived breast cancer only to die years later of ovarian cancer. Her sister is a breast cancer survivor. Her mother carries the BRCA mutation.

Bourn never really questioned having a double mastectomy. It lowered her risk of breast cancer by 90 percent. She also knew she wanted the operation at St. Charles. Both her mother and her sister had double mastectomies there before her. As she did her homework, Bourn could see why her mother and sister chose the facility.

There is simply no other hospital of its kind like it anywhere else.

St. Charles is the only hospital in the world dedicated exclusively for breast cancer surgery and reconstruction. It is the leading medical destination in the United States for breast reconstruction. Its team has performed more than four thousand procedures since its opening in 2009.

It is so well known to women on breast cancer message boards that many just refer to the hospital as NOLA, for the city and state where it resides.

A private, thirty-six-bed licensed hospital, St. Charles is as spalike as a health care facility can be, with towering, light-filled atriums; a chef who customizes meals for patients and caregivers; robes for patients and linens for their overnight guests; and close, individualized nursing care.

The team here pioneered some of the most important breakthroughs in breast reconstruction of the last decade, including nipple-sparing mastectomy and autologous breast reconstruction with a woman's own abdominal, thigh, butt, or back tissue.

"What we view as successful reconstruction is not can it fill a bra or look good in clothes," said Dr. Scott Sullivan, cofounder. "We want patients to get out of the bathtub and love the way they look and not see cancer. Our expectations are high. We want to make it gentle on the body, gentle on the mind, and create an environment that is physically and emotionally conducive to healing. As good as it is here, we are always looking to improve."

Its leading operation, and the gold standard of autologous reconstruction at top centers all over the United States, is what Bourn came for: the Deep Inferior Epigastric Perforator flap, or DIEP. It is a technique that uses a section of abdominal tissue and its connecting deep inferior epigastric vessels to create a new breast, in a method that spares nearby muscle. The St. Charles team offers another half-dozen breast reconstruction techniques with tissue, including a stacked DIEP flap, a gluteal hip flap, and a multiple flap procedure and lift coined the Body Lift flap.

An earlier procedure known as the TRAM flap has fallen in disregard among many plastic surgeons because it takes a larger swath of tissue and muscle, possibly compromising a woman's later ability to bend and reach. It is not performed at St. Charles. "TRAM flaps caused high incidences of hernias and abdominal weakness, even difficulty getting out of bed," said Dr. Whit Wise, one of two microvascular plastic surgeons performing Bourn's procedure. "A DIEP flap saves that muscle entirely."

Most notably, surgery at St. Charles is different from most hospitals, even those with large cancer programs, because it uses two separate teams that work simultaneously on each patient. One team performs the mastectomy portion of the surgery while a second team of microvascular plastic surgeons removes and prepares tissue specimens.

Elsewhere, unless at very large academic institutions or top, high-volume programs, most hospitals only have one board-certified, microvascular plastic surgeon performing a breast reconstruction operation.

The extra doctors cut operation times, speed recovery, and reduce the rate of infections to less than 1 percent of the surgeries performed, Wise said.

The team is so adept at the DIEP flap procedure that many bilateral operations are five to seven hours, compared to seven or eight hours or more at many other places, Wise said. Shorter operating times benefit patient recovery, he said. "The longer the abdominal incision remains open, the higher the risk of bacterial contamination," Wise said. "The quicker you get everything sewn together, the less the chance of an infection. We work against the clock."

St. Charles doctors perform enough reconstruction procedures that doctors are comfortable offering several options that may not be offered to candidates elsewhere, including nipple-sparing mastectomy for women with large or droopy breasts, Sullivan said.

"The consensus is, not here, they are not good candidates for nipple-sparing mastectomy because the blood vessels are inadequate or they have wound-healing issues," Sullivan explained. "In fact, we find it's quite the contrary. The blood vessels are going to be more than adequate. It ends up being a better reconstruction because a woman that size, the largest implant they make for her . . . may look like a little B cup. It may be inadequate. The woman with more tissue, she can be a bigger size. You can cut to fit the volume you need up there." The St. Charles team published a July 2014 report describing their success performing nipple-sparing mastectomy for women with larger or sagging breasts.[1]

⸺◦《◉》◦⸺

Katrina Bourn grew up in a family where women got breast and ovarian cancer. Her grandmother and sister had breast cancer. Her grandmother was diagnosed years later with ovarian cancer and died of it. She and her mother carry the BRCA1 mutation.

She is an example of the growing number of women with extensive family histories of breast and ovarian cancer who are undergoing preventive mastectomies and surgical removal of their ovaries.

The question for many women is not if they will undergo preventive surgery, but when.

Bourn got tested in 2011 after her sister found a lump in her breast while she was breastfeeding her three-month-old child. "I went and met with a geneticist in Baton Rouge and had blood drawn and he called me to tell me I was BRCA1 positive, which increases your risk of breast, ovarian, bile duct, and pancreatic cancers," Bourn said. The test results didn't surprise her, but it was very emotional, she said.

"I immediately started crying," she recalled. "The doctor heard my voice and he stayed on the phone in silence for at least 10 minutes. I composed myself to ask, 'what now?' I had a feeling it was going to be positive but hearing it was a completely different thing."

She was thirty-two at the time; her boys then were two and eight. By having preventive surgery, women can lower a hereditary risk of breast cancer by as much as 90 percent, and by 50 percent for ovarian cancer.

She weighed her options and decided to have a hysterectomy and oophorectomy first to remove her fallopian tubes, uterus, and ovaries. "I already had two children so that was easy," she said. "Still, it was kind of sad. Even though I never wanted more than two children, it was hard to take a step to never be able to have more kids. There's a difference knowing you can if you want to."

Tall with a larger bust and frame, Bourn said she "always wanted a breast reduction but insurance wouldn't pay for it, even though my doctor wrote a note saying it was a medical necessity." The way she looks at it, she would significantly lower her risk of breast cancer with the operation and essentially get a tummy tuck. She reviewed all the reconstruction options and talked to her husband, Tim, whom she's been with since high school. She said he told her, "'Whatever you decide, I'll support you; you do what you need to do for you.' When I found this option, neither one of us could see a down side."

Bourn chose breast reconstruction with her own tissue instead of implants because "it's more like your natural breast. It's still your own body.

It's not like a fake implant with your skin just holding it in there that would be cold to the touch and have no sensation."

Traveling nearly four hours for her surgery came at a cost. Bourn's health insurance covered the surgery but billed it as an out-of-network rate that covered 75 percent of the surgery. Her costs will be about 25 percent of the bill, she said. "There wasn't a point in this journey here that my insurance denied me any service," she said.

The day before her June 3 surgery, Katrina and Tim came to the Center for Restorative Breast Surgery next to St. Charles hospital for her presurgery appointment. The couple thumbed through scrapbooks other patients have created of their surgical stories stretched out on a coffee table in the two-story atrium. A nurse called their names and brought them to an exam room where they met several members of Bourn's team.

The visit, presurgical marking, and CT scans before surgery tied up the Bourns for much of the afternoon.

———— ◉ ————

By 5:30 a.m., Bourn was up and ready for surgery. Nurses started an intravenous line in her arm and took her vital signs. While she waited, members of her surgery team stopped in to review the plan for the operation with her once again. A nurse took down Tim's cell phone number so she could call every hour or two with updates. Here, caregivers don't have to wait until the surgery is over to get news.

Surgery began at 7:02 a.m., and quickly the team split up for their appropriate tasks.

Breast surgeon Dr. Allan Stolier and several other doctors began a mastectomy on Bourn's left breast, cutting or searing away little sections of skin and tissue in a triangular wedge under her breast, while saving her nipple and areola.

At the same time, two microvascular plastic surgeons began making what would become a long hip-to-hip incision about three inches under Bourn's belly button.

"Most places in the country make this incision much higher because it's easier for the doctors," explained Dr. Craig Blum, another microvascular plastic surgeon performing Bourn's operation. "The largest blood vessels are right around the belly button. The problem with making the incision that high is that the bottom incision has to be higher. We want the bottom incision to be very low, so it can be hidden by a bathing suit or your underwear."

Blum said while sparing the muscle attached to the skin flap is time consuming, it helps women retain abdominal strength they would have lost in earlier TRAM procedures. "You make an incision and lift the skin and fat until you see the side of the rectus muscle," he said. "If you open the rectus muscle fibers, opening it like pages in a book, you can see the DIEP vessels. They send up perforator vessels to the skin. That's what we want."

Wise said he and Blum each removed about three-and-a-half-pound flaps from Bourn's right and left abdomen.

"We actually took a little more than that and trimmed it back," he said.

The flaps were removed, placed on a sterile wrap on a nearby surgical table, and were prepared for transfer. First, two assistants must trim the outer layer of skin around the flap one section at a time, ribbon by ribbon. Wise said the process ensured "we don't have any hair follicles or sweat glands under her breast skin." Because the flaps are mostly fat, the tissue can survive for hours without a blood supply, Wise said.

To reduce stomach pain, patients get a few local shots of anesthetic drugs in their abdomen.

On a dry-erase board, the surgery team charted both the amount of tissue, in grams, they removed from both of Bourn's breasts and each side of her abdomen. Each time doctors trimmed additional abdominal fat from the flap, because it was more than what they needed, they subtracted more weight from the chart.

The surgery team now was ready to transfer the section of Bourn's left abdominal tissue to her right breast and her right section to her left breast.

Wise attached additional vessels when one edge of the flap didn't look as healthy. "The more volume you have the more blood supply you need," he explained. "With her, her blood supply was a little inadequate to get to that margin down there. A lot of times you let these recover and they usually recover on their own. Hers is recovering. It's getting pinker and pinker. We don't want a problem so I thought, it's better to adjust it now."

The flaps are transferred in opposite directions. Dr. Chris Trahan, another reconstructive plastic surgeon, explained: "We go left tummy to right chest. We look at the abdominal weight we removed. That's 1,500 grams. Tissue removed from the right breast is 1,165. So to get to where she wants to be we've got to downsize. What we do is we rotate the flap 90 degrees counterclockwise; that's the best part of the flap in terms of fullness. The tip of it here is now up here. We just trimmed it off. Once I get the profusion going, I'm going to look at it and see what I can take off. We'll see how well it performs."

The critical part of the operation is the joining of the internal mammary vessels to the deep epigastric vessels. The internal mammary arteries "are the same blood vessels heart surgeons use for cardiac bypass surgery," Wise said. "They get to them by splitting the sternum. We get to it by lifting a little rib off of it."

Using a high-powered operating microscope, Trahan clamped a tiny plastic coupler device around both vessels he soon would merge. Then he wrapped each with a thin, temporary Doppler wire used to monitor blood flow. He joined the two valves with surgical thread as thin as a human hair.

Operating room staff stopped to see and hear Bourn's reconnected arteries pulse and whir. The temporary Doppler "has a receiver that sends a little signal and lets us monitor things for the first few hours after surgery," Sullivan said. "The artery makes a noise, phew, phew phew. The vein can be variable or make a whir, whir sound or different than that. The venous signal is a little less reliable. For us, this is the most accurate way for us to follow a patient."

"Some people don't use them," Sullivan added. "We find they give us a lot of good data. When we are done listening to them, they slide out real easy. The plastic cup stays but the wire that attaches slides out."

The procedure largely done, Trahan asked registered nurse Don Johnson to take a picture of the connected blood vessels. The photo ensures that the woman got the procedure she requested. Blum said, "Once you close it up, no one knows what goes on underneath there. So it's possible for someone to say they did a DIEP operation when they did more of a TRAM operation."

Trahan added, "At the end of day it's what you leave behind in a patient. Did you spare the muscle or didn't you?"

Trahan called the vessel hookup "a very technically demanding part of the procedure. There's two components. You have to have the skill of a watchmaker to handle really small things, and that's just transferring the tissue. The artistic component is a separate entity. To get it up there is one thing; to get it to look like a breast is another."

Bourn was scheduled to come back in three months for a breast lift. That procedure can't be done at the same time as a nipple-sparing mastectomy, Sullivan said. He explained, "What's going on between now and the second surgery is it's all becoming one. We have the flap growing into the skin and the skin growing into the flap and the chest wall. They are dependent on each other. It's one unit. Now we can mold it and use shaping principles to reconstruct it. We set things up to be successful at this stage. We're shaping the perimeter to get the position on the chest wall right. When you come back for the second stage, the lower number of variables you have to correct the more predictable the result is."

Sullivan drew on a notepad to show how he makes incisions for a breast lift after reconstruction. "When we do a lift for a woman who is really droopy, this is where we make an incision around or even within the areola if you want and we make this triangular incision. In a lift, we take out all this skin, leaving the nipple and areola attached to the underlying tissue. And we push this up and bring the skin edges in and you are left with a scar pattern around the areola and down to the fold."

"She wants to get to a D or DD, which is 700 or 800 grams, we'll put 900 grams in here and close it up. At the second stage we'll do this lift. Little capillaries will grow from the skin and underlying tissue into the flap to help integrate it. When we do her second stage three weeks from now that abdominal fat will have vascularized the skin as well as the breast tissue did. So you can go back and make a small incision around the nipple and areola and take the skin out because the nipple and areola are attached to that abdominal fat. We can do the lift and close it."

"When we talk about whether women are candidates for nipple sparing or not, some limit it to women who are minimally ptotic, with not much droopiness. We'll agree for women with droopiness, they are not the ideal candidate. But you can still do it but in the second stage you do the lift."

"All we did was take out the lower abdominal fat. We've taken off 3,000 grams, about 7 pounds, of tissue. If we were doing a cosmetic tummy tuck, we would take the same amount, with the same closure, a scar down below. And we can do liposuction of the abdomen in the next stage. We don't want to do it now and risk additional blood loss. With additional blood loss, she'd be more prone to hypotension, or low blood pressure, and if the blood pressure is too low the blood vessels will clot up or the tissue will not perfuse well enough."

In the final stage of the operation, Blum took the upper part of Bourn's abdomen and stretched and tightened it downward, covering the old belly button.

Doctors cut the skin around the belly button to expose it again.

———●«❮●❯»●———

Bourn's first day after surgery involved careful monitoring by the nursing staff. "We provide a lot of services for the caregiver as well," said Mikeal Swift, director of nursing. "We think that's important." The hospital allows one overnight visitor to stay with a patient. The guest has a foldout bed and their own linens. A snack bar down the hall often serves as a caregivers' hangout.

"We do a lot of teaching here because there's a lot they need to know when they get home, how to shower, dressings and drains," she said. "It's a whole lot of information and it's too much for one person. We tell the caregiver to get a good night's sleep."

The main goal after the operation is to get women back on their feet and informed about how to take care of themselves for the next few weeks, Swift said. Women leave the hospital with surgical drains she or her caregiver must monitor and keep track of any fluid drainage.

"Then the next morning, our goals are to assess their pain situation, try to wean them off the pain pump, depending how they are doing; get them out of the chair. We try to move our patients early. It prevents complications, leg issues like deep vein thrombosis and respiratory issues. We might try to get them to walk around the room a little bit. The first day is about getting their pain under control. Possibly getting them on oral meds. If we get their pain under control, we can build a trusting relationship and ask them to do a little bit more because they know it's not going to hurt."

"We have oxygen in every room. All the rooms are connected to the nurse's station. They have pain buttons, pumps, the first night. They can't overdo it. They get a set amount each hour. We help them shower from the beginning to the end. It's a new experience. For many, it's the first time they've looked in the mirror. They're exhausted. Their body has been through a lot."

"We provide toiletries, blow driers, robes. They can put on their own pajamas after they shower. They like to wear something that buttons down the front because we will be checking them frequently."

By day two postop, women are encouraged to move around the room or walk the halls. Day three, typically, is discharge, with strict restrictions on many activities, including lifting anything more than ten pounds for six weeks.

Bourn was home five days later. She developed an infection in one nipple and risked losing it. It came around after five rounds of antibiotics. The nipple "is healing well," Bourn said, in a mid-August 2015 email. "I've started driving again, working from home and exercising. I'm pretty much all-clear on return to all activities."

Her plan was to return in December 2015 for a breast lift and tuneup procedure, as most women do.

7

Silicone Implants

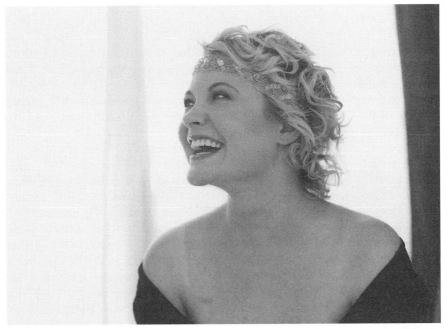

Emmy Pontz-Rickert had breast cancer surgery at age twenty-four. Two years later, she gave birth to a baby girl.

Just twenty-four when she was diagnosed with breast cancer in March 2013, Emily Pontz-Rickert, a legislative aide to a Michigan state senator, felt compelled to move quickly.

She had an aggressive, triple-negative breast cancer.

Because of delays getting the results of genetic testing, Pontz-Rickert decided to get going with a single mastectomy only to find out she carried the BRCA2 gene mutation that greatly raises her risk of breast and ovarian cancer. The results made her choose to remove her other breast and undergo silicone breast reconstruction after she finished chemotherapy eight months later.

"For me it was the easiest decision," said Pontz-Rickert, enjoying her life as a full-time mother, as well as an activist for breast cancer groups and an African children's foundation. "I just wanted to be done. I wanted to move on with my life."

Breast reconstruction with silicone implants is by far the most common type of breast reconstruction performed in the United States. And it almost always has been, except for a fourteen-year period from January 1992 to November 2006, when the federal Food and Drug Administration placed a moratorium on their use because of safety issues.[1]

Of 102,215 reconstruction procedures performed in 2014 in the United States, 77,080 used silicone implants, an 11 percent increase from the year before.[2]

Recovery is considered easier and quicker than tissue reconstruction, though corrections and revisions can keep women going back to their plastic surgeons for months, and even years. A major reason for the preference is that more plastic surgeons perform reconstruction with implants than with tissue-based methods, which require more extensive training and expertise.

"I came to work here in 1989, almost immediately when the implant controversy began," recalled Dr. Edwin Wilkins, professor of plastic surgery at the University of Michigan. "We providers and the patients were all scared senseless that the silicone gel we had been using was suddenly a danger to people's health. If you are a surgeon, that's a nightmare thinking you may have hurt some patients. I thought maybe I should stick with saline and avoid any possible problem. The problem was my results suffered, to be quite honest. They were not as good as they could have been or should have been. So by 2003 or 2004 I had patients in whom I put expanders and we started talking about the exchange operations. They asked for silicone gel. Then they asked to be referred to plastic surgeons who used gel. I essentially was pushed back into using silicone gel. When I did, I felt kind of foolish I hadn't done it sooner. The results are clearly better, especially in thinner women. There's so much less visible wrinkling and they have a softer texture. Saline has a tense, water-balloon-like texture whereas a silicone implant, unless they encapsulate, are nice, soft and doughy."

Today's implants usually are implanted in a two-step process at the time of mastectomy, using a temporary device or expander that doctors fill with salt water in stages to stretch the chest skin to hold an implant. Usually, implants are placed below the chest muscle.

IMPLANT PLACEMENT IN ATHLETIC WOMEN

For years, plastic surgeons have preferred to place breast implants under the main muscle in the chest.

But younger, athletic women having preventive mastectomies, and some plastic surgeons have begun to challenge that conventional wisdom.

If a woman is very athletic or lifts weights, some plastic surgeons believe she is better off having what doctors call prepectoral placement of the implant. The method is used with additional cadaver and animal tissue known as acellular dermal matrix products, or ADM.

The discussion emerged at the annual conference in 2015 in Philadelphia of Facing Our Risk of Cancer Empowered, or FORCE. Women asked about the issue at several of the conference's surgery sessions, which included a leading speaker on the subject.

Dr. Hilton Becker, a Boca Raton, Florida, plastic surgeon, said he has performed prepectoral implant placement for about seven years, after seeing too many patients develop distortions in their implants when they exercised or the devices moved too high up on their chests. He calls the first problem "animation distortion" and the second "high-riding implants."

He uses an adjustable saline implant that can be filled with saltwater in stages. He also adds an ADM product to hold the implant in place, over the muscle.

When the implant is filled to the desired size of the breast, Becker takes out a tiny valve from the implant and closes up the site. Sometimes, he swaps the temporary saline implant for a silicone one, for women interested in the more natural look they think silicone provides. He said adjustable gel implants are available in Europe and many other regions, but not the United States.

Dr. Scott Spear, a Chevy Chase, Maryland, plastic surgeon, said he has seen doctors change attitudes on the subject, but he urged caution about the placement of implants.

Doctors usually place implants under the pectoral muscle because they will be "less noticeable, more protectable," he said. The addition of ADM products on top of an implant also will change the look of an implant, he said. "It's not going to look as soft." He said women should raise the issue with their plastic surgeons if they are very athletic.

"If someone came to me and said they were really worried about the animation thing and they were worried about lifting weights, I'd do a prepectoral placement."

Dr. Steven Kronowitz, a professor of plastic surgery at the University of Texas MD Anderson Cancer Center, Houston, said the placement of implants above the chest muscle makes it harder to find suspicious areas on mammograms. "We can see more of the breast tissue during a mammogram when the implant is below the muscle, making it easier to detect changes," he said.

While some women tolerate the expander portion of reconstruction, others find it the most painful part of the process.

"The expanders are extremely uncomfortable," said Belinda Cox, an archeologist who lives in Ashville, North Carolina, talking in April 2015 as she neared completion of the expander phase of reconstruction. "I don't sleep. I've been sleeping on the couch since my last fill up. I keep my partner awake. It's really full and painful, the size of a grapefruit. The nurse jokes she could put a dinner plate on it. Yep, that puppy is full." Because of these problems, some doctors offer a one-step implant procedure that does not require expanders.

ONE-STEP IMPLANT RECONSTRUCTION

Dr. C. Andrew Salzberg, a Tarrytown, New York, plastic surgeon, developed one-step breast implant reconstruction in 2000.

He heard so many women complain about the expander phase of silicone breast implant reconstruction that he decided to do something about it, he said.

The direct-to-implant breast reconstruction approach allows doctors to do implant reconstruction without the so-called two-step process of expanders, temporary, adjustable saline devices used to stretch the skin to hold an implant.

Direct-to-implant reconstruction is done with acelullar dermal matrix, or ADM, products made from human and pig skin, stripped of everything but a collagen layer, then sterilized. Doctors use thin layers of ADM products to support an implant and to add contour to the breast.

The methods are called direct-to-implant, single-stage breast reconstruction with acellular dermal matrix.

Usually, direct-to-implant reconstruction is performed with a nipple-sparing mastectomy. It is a good option for younger, thinner women undergoing preventive mastectomies.

Larger, bustier women, and even some women who have had prior chest radiation, also may be able to have a one-step procedure as long as they do not have extremely droopy breasts and their breast skin is healthy enough to hold an implant immediately, Salzberg said, describing the approach to the 2015 annual meeting of FORCE, a large hereditary cancer organization.

Salzberg uses a dye, injected into the breast skin, to see if it is healthy. "If the skin is good, we proceed," he said. If the skin doesn't look healthy enough, conventional reconstruction with expanders may be necessary, he said.

Salzberg said he followed 692 patients over fourteen years that have had direct-to-implant reconstruction. The data show that one-step reconstruction is effective, with a rate of capsular contracture, a hardening of the implant, occurring less than 1 percent of the time. Overall, 96 percent of patients had no postoperative complications; 9.4 percent needed at least a second revision surgery, mostly to get their breasts to match better.

Other studies of direct-to-implant methods with ADM have found the approach effective, particularly in smaller women. In one study published in 2014, Dr. Perry Gdalevitch, a Vancouver, British Columbia, plastic surgeon, concluded, "Direct-to-implant reconstruction can be reliably performed in a single stage in patients with small breast size. Increasing breast size confers a higher chance of early revision." The team found the approach more successful in preventive mastectomies; smoking and breast size increased a woman's chance of problems.

For now, doctors continue to work on figuring out who is the best candidate for one-stage reconstruction. "You need to have several factors for it to work," said Dr. Joseph Disa, a plastic surgeon at New York City's Memorial Sloan Kettering Cancer Center. He said he performs the approach in about 10 percent of his reconstruction cases. First, he explains two critical factors, he said.

"The patient needs to want a new breast that is their current size or a little bit smaller. Number two. Their breasts can't be too big. The bigger the breast, the higher the reconstructive failure. So you want small-to-moderate-sized breasts in a woman who wants to be the same size or smaller. She's the best candidate. And the final issue is the breast surgeon who does the mastectomy. It's critical the skin flaps have adequate blood flow and are of adequate thickness to make that operation work. If the skin flaps are ischemic or have poor blood flow or they are very thin and they won't tolerate the weight of an implant, then it's not going to work."

REFLECTIONS FROM ONE-STEP IMPLANT PATIENT

Dr. Elizabeth Thompson, forty-six, of Scarsdale, New York, was one of the first women in America to have a direct-to-implant double mastectomy, in 2006.

Dr. C. Andrew Salzberg and Dr. Andrew Ashikari, her surgery team, were among the pioneers of the procedure. Direct-to-implant or one-stage implant reconstruction inserts silicone implants at the time of a mastectomy, without the use of temporary expanders.

Thompson recovered easily from the procedure. She returned to running twelve days later and went on with her busy life as a mother of four and a radiation oncologist.

A year later, she needed a revision procedure to help her breasts match better, but otherwise, her implants gave her a lasting choice. "For me, my body is pretty much the same except for the loss of sensation in most of my breast and nipples," she said. "If you are not OK with that, you need to talk to your partner about it because it might impact your sex life. I'm happy because I confident I'm not going to get breast cancer. I might get something else but not breast cancer. That's what really scared me."

Thompson had a preventive double mastectomy even though her family's tests showed no known cancer gene mutation. Usually, this type of finding of undetermined significance, as it is called, is treated as a negative result.

But Thompson knew her family's cancer history. "My maternal great-grandmother, grandmother, and mother all had breast cancer," she said.

"Although my mother and I actually test negative for the BRCA mutation, as an oncologist, I suspected there is some other gene that runs in our DNA we just haven't identified yet. As a physician, I already knew too much and I wanted to be proactive. I felt like I had a ticking time bomb in my body. When I told my friends about my upcoming procedure, some of them looked at me like I was crazy, like it was a brutal mutilation. They told me to just wait and see what happens, but I told them the idea of getting the breast cancer diagnosis and having chemo was something I couldn't face. Maybe I was a coward, but I felt like at that point I still had a choice."

She had the testing because "I wanted to be alive and well for my children. So for peace of mind, I heard about a new procedure very close to where I live. Two doctors were pioneering the direct-to-implant reconstruction technique. I researched it. I was patient no. 50. I had a pretty smooth recovery. After that, the physicians asked me to come and work for them with patients, really as a navigator. So when a woman came in for the procedure, I'd talk to them about what I went through, and to prepare them for the hospital and the home. That's where I learned about all the things that were missing in the recovery process. The little things you need that nobody pulled together. I made lists of things the patients would need. It finally became a kit." Thompson went on to make a surgical bra, now patented, that holds drainage tubes she and others find annoying. The bra and the kit are available through her company's website, www.bfflco.com.

Breast implants are not lifetime devices, the FDA warns on its website. "The longer a woman has them, the greater the chances that she will develop complications, some of which will require more surgery."[3] Like saline implants, silicone implants may cause wrinkling or get hard as rocks, a problem known as capsular contracture. After ten to twenty years, the silicone from gel implants can leak and the implants must be removed, as did 17,496 women in 2014 who had undergone implant reconstruction, according to the American Society of Plastic Surgery.[4] The organization, the largest one in the field, has extensive videos and information on its website, http://www.plasticsurgery.org.

Some ruptures, however, that are described as silent go undetected, when silicone gel or silicone oil from the implant may leak out inside the scar tissue, or escape the scar tissue into the breast or surrounding tissue. Because the gel usually leaks slowly, the change in size or shape is often not obvious, so the women will be unaware of the leak unless it causes granulomas, or small lumps consisting of silicone surrounded by scar tissue, or pain. Saline implants can also rupture or leak, but when that happens the leaking saline does not usually cause any problems other than deflating the implant.

The FDA, which regulates implants as a medical device, warns the following on its website, http://www.fda.gov.[5]

- Breast implants are not lifetime devices. The longer a woman has them, the more likely she is to have complications and need to have the implants removed or replaced. Women with breast implants will need to monitor their breasts for the rest of their lives.
- The most frequently observed complications and adverse outcomes are tightening of the area around the implant (capsular contracture), additional surgeries, and implant removal. Other complications include a tear or hole in the outer shell (implant rupture), wrinkling, uneven appearance (asymmetry), scarring, pain, and infection.

- Women with implants lose sensation in their breasts.
- Studies to date do not indicate that silicone-gel-filled breast implants cause breast cancer, reproductive problems, or connective tissue disease, such as rheumatoid arthritis. However, no study has been large enough or long enough to completely rule out these and other rare complications.

The FDA has more information on implant issues, questions to ask doctors, and several videos, at http://www.fda.gov.

Manufacturers say new types of implants are tougher and safer than the previous generations of implants.

Silicone implants come in various shapes and textured surfaces, such as round or tear-dropped or textured or smooth. But the biggest change in the last decade has been in the type of silicone used inside the latest implants.

Highly cohesive gel implants are also called gummy bear implants and are anatomically shaped. "They have a more viscous, thicker gel, more of a jelly, or the proverbial gummy bear," said Dr. Michael Meininger, a Birmingham, Michigan, plastic surgeon who has been part of studies for the devices. "It holds its shape. The old gels were like honey and when the bag broke it went everywhere. The new ones are cohesive and sticky, more like peanut butter. You can cut a hole in it and the stuff won't bulge out. In the fifth generation, we'd shape the skin with a tissue expander. Then we'd put in the round implant and we'd hope the shaped skin could hold that round implant. Sometimes it did, sometimes it didn't. These new implants are actually oval. So you can customize them for the east, north, south, and west dimension and you can customize them for projection. They come in so many shapes that they can be used to match the mastectomy defect with more consistency."

Dr. Dennis Hammond, a Grand Rapids, Michigan, plastic surgeon and national speaker on implants and a consultant to several implant companies, also finds that anatomical implants retain their shape and are less prone to wrinkles or capsular contracture. "The anatomic gel implant has the best safety profile of them all," he said. "Tissue expanders allow you to do the reconstruction in one place without making additional incisions in the body," he said, referring to tissue-based reconstruction.

Other experts consider the jury still out on the new implants. Some aren't convinced, citing issues with movement of the implants if the pocket created during the mastectomy is not form fitting or tight enough to hold the implant so it will not shift.

"In unilateral cases, there's no question patients benefit from an anatomically shaped device," said Dr. Jesse Selber, a plastic surgeon at Houston's MD Anderson Cancer Center.

"For the bilateral patient, there are a lot of considerations, including the shape of the chest wall, the height of the breast, and the projection of the breast," Selber said. "The round device gives a little bit of a different, rounder look. The anatomical devices have a more sloping upper pole. In Europe, where they are a bit more conservative, in terms of everything that has to do with the breast, they have been using these devices for a long time. I've been happy with the aesthetics. Americans are kind of a little behind them on that, I'd say."

Others, including Wilkins and Diana Zuckerman, PhD, a scientist who has studied the safety of breast implants since initiating congressional hearings on the topic in 1990, await more studies.

"The 50-year history of breast implants is the history of repeated claims that the newest silicone implants are safer," said Zuckerman, president of the National Center for Health Research and founder of its Cancer Prevention and Treatment Fund, a Washington, D.C.–based nonprofit think tank with a breast implant website, http://www.breastimplantinfo.org.

"When 'gummy bear' implants are new, you can cut them with a knife and they don't leak but that doesn't mean that after three or more years in the human body, at 98.6 degrees and warmer, the silicone gel is not going to break down in some way like other breast implants," Zuckerman said.

"The very first breast implants in this country sold in the 1960s were a very, very thick gel," she added. "Those implants did last longer than the ones that replaced them in the 1970s, which were too thin. But even those original thick gel implants did eventually leak, break, and cause problems. There are no studies to let women know which implants are safer or which last longer. There have been no long-term studies in the United States of gummy bear implants, beyond about a six-year study. Six years doesn't tell you very much, since most safety issues arise after 10–15 years. Our center is already hearing from many women who have had terrible problems with their gummy bear implants. It wouldn't surprise me if plastic surgeons over the years find that these newer implants may not be any safer than the earlier breast implants."

———————

Emily Pontz-Rickert was pleased with her silicone implant reconstruction. But the process didn't go as smoothly as she wanted, right from the start. Her story illustrates how important it is for some women to have breasts and the issues many encounter getting them.

She found a lump in her breast as she fiddled with a necklace one day at work, she said. She might otherwise have ignored it, but her aunt Jody had just died of breast cancer.

"Normally at 24 I never would have thought this was breast cancer but with my aunt's death from breast cancer I went to my ob-gyn the next day," she said. She remembered the doctor saying, "I do feel something but you are so young so it's not going to be anything serious. But just in case, I want you to get an ultrasound. They also said, 'you are so young we're really not too worried about it. But just in case, you need a biopsy.' At that point, my gut was telling me it was something bad. I knew at that point I might have breast cancer."

"Three days later on March 18, the doctor called me on his cell phone while he was on vacation. I knew then it wasn't good news. I was at work. He said, 'I'm so surprised I'm calling you right now. I need to tell you that you have breast cancer and it's a very aggressive form of breast cancer' known as a triple-negative breast cancer." These tumors lack estrogen, progesterone, and protein targets on breast cells that chemotherapy attacks.

Within two weeks, in March 2013, Pontz-Rickert underwent a unilateral mastectomy without reconstruction because she was waiting for the results of genetic testing her doctors suggested she have because of her young age. The test results, which did not arrive in time for her first surgery, found that she had a BRCA2 gene mutation and made her change her mind and have a double mastectomy. But she would have to finish chemotherapy first.

She called the months living one-breasted her "uni-boob stage." She refused to wear a prosthesis or wig when her hair fell out from chemotherapy. "I chose to rock the bald, as I called it," she said.

She also grew to feel empowered by her scar. "I decided I was really glad I had the scar for the time I did but I don't want to let it win over the rest of my life," she said at the time. "I want to be able to wear a bathing suit again. I want to look beautiful in my wedding dress the day I get married. I want to feel beautiful for my husband. I don't want people to look at me and say, 'look, she must have had cancer or something.'"

She arranged with a friend, a professional photographer, to take photographs of her, exposing her mastectomy scar, which she has donated to several cancer centers, including the Susan P. Wheatlake Cancer Center in Reed City, Michigan, and the Betty Ford Cancer Center at Spectrum Hospital, Grand Rapids, Michigan. "My scars show strength," she said. "The photos prove that cancer didn't beat me."

Before starting chemotherapy in May, a friend of Pontz-Rickert created a http://www.gofundme.com account through the internet fund-raising site to raise money so she could afford to freeze her eggs for possible use someday in an in-vitro fertilization procedure. "It was difficult but it gave me such hope," she said. "For me, my number-one fear has been hoping and making sure I can have children."

Unfortunately, the worse was to come. "Chemotherapy affects everyone differently," she said. "I was one of the ones it really knocked down.

It was awful. I was literally in bed pretty much unconscious to the world for a week and a half. I don't remember anything in that week and a half. I thought chemo probably would be the easiest because I had gone through so much already. But really, it was kind of the nail in the coffin. I'm still dealing with major side effects. Your immune system is shot."

The drug cytoxan gave her a "bad bladder infection." Even two antibiotics didn't work, and she required hospitalization when she developed a severe kidney infection. Another chemotherapy drug, taxotere, caused pain "all over my body, kind of like what fibromyalgia patients go through, especially in the morning, I was so stiff in the morning, I could barely get out of bed." Another drug, Lupron, that she took to keep her ovaries from making estrogen "gave me horrible hot flashes."

Her weight ballooned during chemotherapy to 148 pounds, up from 120 pounds. Then she gathered her strength up for another mastectomy, this time to remove her healthy breast and begin reconstruction with expanders. Her doctors also used an ADM product to shape and shore up the implants.

Like many women, she found the expander phase of reconstruction difficult. "I have good days and bad days," she said, nearing the end of the filler process at the time. "I'm less than a week from my implant surgery. I am extremely sore. Yesterday, actually, I passed out at work and threw up and I was taken home because of the pain in my chest. I think the expanders will be worth it in the end, but they have been less than comfortable. I just kind of count down the days until my implant surgery. I can't wait. It's the end of this very long, hard process. The light at the end of the tunnel."

In September 2014, Pontz-Rickert got news that more than offset her treatment challenges. She and her husband, Kelly Rickert, were expecting a baby, without having to have an IVF procedure. "Kelly and I began trying to conceive right away," Pontz-Rickert said. "We were thinking two things: If I can't conceive, we will need time to do IVF or adoption. And it will take forever to naturally conceive if that is even possible."

"We actually conceived the very night we started trying. For me, it was God's way of telling me, good job my child. You have survived the worst and experienced great sadness in your short lifetime. Here is the happiest gift I can give you."

Grace Angelin was born in May 15, 2015. "She is truly our rainbow at the end of a storm. A true miracle." She added, "We hope to have a few more before my preventive oophorectomy at approximately age 32."

Pontz-Rickert continues seeing her medical oncologist for tests and checkups. She undergoes CA-125 blood tests for ovarian cancer. She plans to eventually have surgery to remove her ovaries, fallopian tubes, and uterus, but for now, that has to wait. She and her husband want more children, and she savors her new life as a full-time homemaker, with projects on the side helping breast cancer groups and Hope for Huruma, a children's home and school in Kenya.

She is sad she can't breastfeed her new baby, but she found another benefit of reconstruction. "My results, although unfinished, still awaiting nipples, look wonderful," said Pontz-Rickert. "My clothing fits normally, which I know those with mastectomies would understand is very nice." However, she added, "I struggle greatly with the fact that I cannot breast-feed. It tears at my heart daily. I actually always looked forward to and idealized breastfeeding. I know other young women probably will go through this feeling, and I want them to know that it is shared and very normal."

But having breasts gave her an unexpected benefit that greatly pleased her. She loves to cradle her baby. "I really appreciate them because my chest, instead of being all bones, is comfortable for my baby to sleep soundly on." However, by February 2016, her implants had become pain-ful. Pontz-Rickert had them removed, she told friends on her Facebook page.

8

Saline Implants

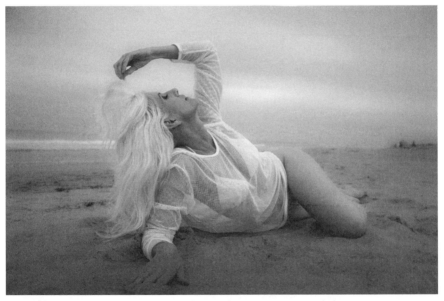

Marjorie Hacker, who remembers the implant controversy of the 1990s, says, "No silicone in this tata."

Marjorie Hacker quickly made her reconstruction choice when she was diagnosed with breast cancer.

She was too thin for surgery to create a new breast with her own tummy, buttock, thigh, or other tissue, and she didn't want to risk damaging a muscle, a possible complication of some tissue-transfer procedures, she said.

She picked saline, or saltwater-filled breast implants, what she considered then and she still believes are the safest breast reconstruction option. She still has her original pair, and she's happy with them.

At the time Hacker had her procedure in 2005, a federal ban on silicone implants limited nearly all women to saline implants, while safety issues were under study.

Hacker, fifty-two, of Boynton Beach, Florida, remembers congressional implant hearings where women testified about serious health problems they and their doctors attributed to silicone implants. "No silicone in this tata," said Hacker, a yoga instructor. "Why would I ever get silicone? If it did pop in my body, at least it would be water."

The federal ban of silicone implants, started in 1992, was lifted in 2006 after studies demanded by the federal Food and Drug Administration of implant manufacturers cleared silicone of long-term health problems.

Quickly, silicone returned as the implant preference in the United States. For every twelve women who get silicone implants, only one picks saline.

In 2014, 6,069 American women had reconstruction with saline implants, compared to 77,080 women who chose silicone, according to the American Society of Plastic Surgeons.[1]

Plastic surgeons and implant manufacturers say newer silicone models available in the United States in the last few years give women more options. They come in larger sizes and shapes, including styles that give more projection, as well as fullness, in the lower portion of the breast. These products create more options for larger-breasted women. Silicone also more closely replicates the look of a natural breast, some plastic surgeons say, besides being more durable and less prone to exterior wrinkling than saline.

"I have a preference that if a patient wants an anatomically shaped implant, she is better off with silicone than with saline because silicone anatomically shaped implants hold their shape better than a saline implant," said Dr. Joseph Disa, a plastic surgeon at New York City's Memorial Sloan Kettering Cancer Center.

Still, saline implants have their benefits. If they break, they only leak water. They also can give women and their plastic surgeons more leeway in deciding the final size of their breasts, an issue many women struggle with, said Dr. Karen Horton, a San Francisco plastic surgeon.

Horton uses a saline implant with a small port, or injection dome, that allows her to make a breast implant smaller or bigger depending on a woman's preference and ability to retain a larger implant.

Horton explained it this way: "When I joined this practice eight years ago, my former partner, Loren Eskenazi, developed a technique I've since adopted, which is to use a permanent saline implant from Mentor Corp. called the Spectrum implant.[2] What's different about it is that it has a smooth wall, as opposed to texture. It's a permanent implant with a remote port. It's put in the tissue where the breast was, not under the chest muscle. We put it on top of the muscle in the space where the breast used to be. That makes sense to me because that's where we are missing tissue. With that injection dome, we can modify the implant volume to suit the patient's goals. They can decide as the swelling goes down, oh, do I look beautiful or do I want them a little bigger? The nice thing is, when they are happy with the size, three to four weeks after surgery, then we let everything sit because it takes about three months or so for most of the surgical swelling to go away. At the three-month period, we have a conversation. Are you happy with the size? Do we like the result of the saline implant? If the answer is yes, all I need to do is open part of the scar and remove the port. There's a self-sealing valve that goes off. It's amazing. It gives the patient control. It's been around 35 years. If we are worried there is too much volume in there, putting pressure on the skin, we can remove it after surgery."

Horton also likes the fact that saline implants give women more options than silicone if they need subsequent radiation or chemotherapy, an emerging issue as more women get radiation for aggressive tumors. "Radiation can increase the risk of implant complications like capsular contracture," she explained. "If they develop some contracture while having radiation or in the six-month period afterwards, because that port is in place, if the implant begins to feel tight, we can adjust the volume. It really gives a woman control over her reconstructive outcome."

Saline implants contain sterile, saltwater fluid enclosed within a more solid silicone shell. Like silicone implants, they come in different styles, projections, and sizes. The exterior silicone shell around a saline implant may be round or textured—a type of cross-linking of chemical bonds that aims to make an implant more durable. At the present, whether a woman gets a smooth or textured surface is largely a matter of physician choice. There is some ongoing research about the difference between the two.

The federal Food and Drug Administration, which regulates breast implants, does not recommend that women with saline breast implants have more expensive magnetic resonance imaging, or MRI, tests to detect rupture because saline implants deflate when they leak.

But saline implants have many of the same problems associated with silicone implants, plus some unique issues of their own.

Like silicone, saline implants may interfere with breastfeeding and mammograms, requiring extra mammography views, according to implant manufacturers. They also can break and leak, turn rock hard, or cause an infection. Problems vary with each implant; manufacturers list safety data on their websites. Studies by implant manufacturer Mentor, a California company, for example, show that 41 percent of women with saline implants have a reoperation within three years and 26.8 percent had to have the implant removed.[3] Other companies report similar findings.

The four most common reasons for reoperations for saline implants are: personal reasons, typically to improve appearance; hardening of scar tissue around the implant, a problem known as capsular contracture; leakage; and wrinkling, according to Mentor data.

Breast cancer message boards and websites mention other objections to saline, though these issues aren't well studied either. Problems women report, according to http://www.breastimplantinfo.org, a popular site with breast implant information, include concerns that the "salt-water implant doesn't warm up the way a natural breast does, so their breasts feel cool rather than warm," the site says. "The implants can get unpleasantly cold in very cold weather, according to women who like ice-skating and similar sports. Women with saline implants also complain that the implants may make a swooshing water noise that makes them feel self-conscious."

Hacker has had none of those problems after her double mastectomy. She still has her original saline implants. "No, they don't slosh," she said, when asked. "They are firm. I went hiking in Colorado and I didn't feel like, ooh, I'm going to take off. Maybe if I had picked bigger ones, I would have," she said, laughing.

Hacker, a self-employed artist of pet portraits, was diagnosed with a type of early, noninvasive form of breast cancer known as ductal carcinoma in situ, or DCIS. While contained within her breast, it was scattered throughout "like popcorn had gone off," Hacker explained. She had chemotherapy first, then a single mastectomy and breast lift, or mastopexy, with implant reconstruction so her breasts would match. Two different-sized saline implants were used, as the left breast without cancer had no mastectomy defect like her right one did, so it only needed a smaller implant.

Her left breast still has a nipple and areola, saved during the implant procedure. Her right breast has no nipple or areola. Hacker never went back to have her nipple reconstructed or tattooed because she wasn't convinced the work would look real. "I haven't seen any that are phenomenal," she said of nipple tattoos. None of this bothers James, her partner of fifteen years, who has been supportive throughout.

Overall, she loves her new breasts and thinks "they are fabulous." Still, they aren't her old breasts by far, she said.

"I used to love my little, small, normal-sized breasts," she said. "They were my breasts. Kind of sports titties. Now my breasts are hard but not hard like a rock. I just don't have feeling in my right breast. It really hasn't come back. I just don't feel anything sexual about them. Because there's no enjoyment with them anymore and I wish somebody told me that. You know, I wish somebody would have said your breasts won't have the feeling of your natural breasts. It's not like a regular breast. You can't manipulate it. They look good in clothing."

Hacker doesn't mind giving others a look at her reconstructed breasts. She's a go-to woman in the West Palm Beach, Florida, area. She gets calls every few weeks from newly diagnosed women. She tells it like it is, the good, the bad, the what's behind, the what's ahead.

"Women need to know that breasts can change with age and weight loss or gain," she said. "When you gain or lose weight, the mastectomy breast never loses weight. Only the unaffected breast gains or loses weight. It's something to really think about. My plastic surgeon asked me, is this your normal weight? I can notice it but it's incremental. But if you are a large lady and through lymphedema or whatever, your one breast gets bigger and the other one stays the same."

Since her diagnosis, Hacker has given up meat and fish, diet pop, and frozen foods. "Disease is a way of telling you something's not working, something's not right, and it's a wake-up call," she said. "Either you listen to it or you hide your head in the sand."

9

Flat or One-Breasted

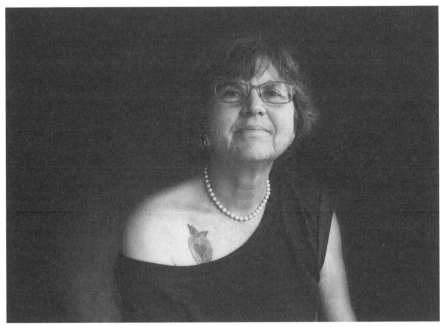

Ann Fonfa has lived both one-breasted and then flat-breasted.

Ann Fonfa likes to share advice with the online Facebook sisterhood, Flat & Fabulous, where women tell their stories or ask questions about decisions to go flat or one-breasted after breast cancer surgery.

The oldest choice of them all, going flat-chested or one-breasted, has new, public support among women making the choice to go unreconstructed.

Facebook groups like Flat & Fabulous in the United States, http://www.flatandfabulous.org, and Flat Friends in the United Kingdom, http://www.flatfriends.org.uk, give support and advice from women who have chosen to rock the boat and say enough after a lumpectomy or mastectomy.

The support groups are much appreciated, women say, because given all the options for breast reconstruction, too many doctors, friends, and others sometimes pressure women to consider reconstruction.

"Sweet Jesus," said Johanna Littleton, forty-four, a middle school reading teacher in Meridian, Mississippi. "Starting with the oncologist. When he told me I should have a mastectomy, the first words out of his mouth were, 'and I'm going to give you the name of a plastic surgeon and he will help with reconstruction.' I told him I wasn't sure what we're going to do. My husband and I don't make rash decisions when it comes to my health. He said, 'well, you are too young. You really need to look at reconstruction.'"

"I don't even talk to my sister now because of all of this," she added. "She made jokes about the whole upgrade, trade-em-in for a bigger pair. My friends at first made light of it. Work colleagues talked to me extensively about reconstruction and why I didn't want to reconstruct. I guess if you have not been through it, you don't get it. All I'm saying is it needs to be on the menu."

Fonfa, Littleton, and three other women who chose not to undergo breast reconstruction explain what it's like living in a breast-conscious world without a set of breasts.

—————————=«(◊)»=—————————

Ann Fonfa, sixty-six, is a speaker at many national conferences on cancer and complementary medicine. In 1999, six years after she was diagnosed with breast cancer, she founded the online Annie Appleseed Project, a nonprofit that offers resources and an annual conference about holistic cancer options. It has a website, http://www.annieappleseedproject.org, that claims more than thirteen million visitors.

Fonfa has lived both one-breasted and flat-chested. Her cancer returned after several lumpectomies and two mastectomies at separate times in each of her breasts. She refused radiation and chemotherapy because she has chemical sensitivities and is an antinuclear war activist who considers radiation harmful. "I wanted a more natural route. Lots of things contributed to my choices."

She had no problem being one-breasted after her first mastectomy, she said. "The first mastectomy was not going to be a problem," she said. "I was a warrior woman. I had got a prosthesis but it weighed so much I didn't wear it much. I never bought the appropriate bra. I donated it to India, where I understand that they cut it in half for two."

"My husband was wonderful about it. We had a long talk on the day of my first mastectomy and he said I had the greatest legs in the world. He switched from being a breast man at that moment. And we both agreed that having safe breasts for me was more important than having a place for sexual action. And I was a bit sensitive."

A diagnosis with Paget's disease, a rare cancer of the nipple or areola that she found around the nipple in her noncancerous breast, led to a second mastectomy. That was tough for her. "After my second mastectomy, I thought, I look like a little boy. I cried about losing my womanhood."

Her breasts, in fact, had been one of her best assets. "I had a D cup," she said. "I developed breasts when I was 10. It was the first thing that ever attracted people to me. I had a large chest. My mother did too. It's what I identified as very attractive about myself as I got older. And they were extremely sensitive in a sexual kind of way."

A walk in New York City, where she once lived, helped her gain clarity about living flat-chested, and she got back her sexier vibe. "I was wearing a tight-fitting spandex kind of top. A gay man walked past me in Manhattan and he looked at me and said, nice bod, so I got over it."

She still has scars, is prone to lymphedema, has a swollen arm and a chest pain problem, and wore compression arm garments until two years ago, when her acupuncturist asked if she could go without it to increase the blood flow on the left. She attributes the relief to her relentless diet and exercise regimen.

After her scars healed, she got the first of several chest tattoos.

"Over time, the scars have gotten better," she said. "They have aged. I discovered my left rib cage was more prominent than the right. I had a couple of tattoos done in 1999. The first one was a full nipple. But I wasn't clear enough to the tattoo artist and I got a little boy's nipple. Then I had a gold-ring tattoo put in for the year of my diagnosis. I thought I might put in a ring for every year I survived. After a while it got painful so I said the heck with that."

"The year after that, I put a snake in it. I love snakes. I had a fighting snake to deal with the cancer. I had another kind of snake put on my shoulder. I asked the tattoo artist to put in the initials SRW. When people asked me what that was, I said, 'those are my husband's initials.' There was shocked silence. When I said, 'those are my lover's initials,' people would say, 'wow, cool.' I told my husband, 'I can always say it means sexually responsive woman.' Last year, I had the logo for my organization put onto my right shoulder."

Left-sided tenderness created bedroom humor between Fonfa and her husband of twenty-seven years. "We joked that he was directionally challenged because he couldn't remember which breast he could touch. We had some confusion."

"When I had my first lumpectomy, I was still lifting up my shirt to flash him. But when I had the mastectomy, he said, 'I can't look at the scar right away.' I stopped showing him my chest. It was quite a while before I did it again. When we moved six years after the surgery to Florida, he said, 'Wow, this is great. Look at the shower.' We have a big shower and we can shower together. Overall, he switched his allegiance. He's fine with it. He must have told me a million times that I was the most beautiful woman in the world and he loved me very much. He's very romantic and very verbal."

"It was important because you need some appreciation when you have such a different look."

She tells other women that living without breasts "over time, it becomes less important. It's just who I am. I have not had reconstruction and I'm fine with it. When I am talking to women who are trembling on the brink, they are thrilled because they have a role model and they can see their life is fine with their choice."

"So my philosophy always has been, you get yourself well. You are about to go through heavy-duty treatment. It's almost like torture. But you know, suffering doesn't always have to be part of it. I recognized it pretty early on. Because of my chemical sensitivity, I did not take chemotherapy. In my support group, everybody was so sick, and I wasn't. I started thinking about getting healthier. I was having more fruits and vegetables, exercising more and taking dietary supplements. I started to get healthier, stronger and more able to deal with cancer. Treatment in the conventional world crushes you."

With her nonprofit, she takes her message to several dozen conferences a year where she is known as an outspoken questioner. "I am the queen of asking, 'why didn't you mention the adverse effects?'"

Her extensive traveling requires ingenuity to keep a healthy, vegan diet. Sometimes, she mails herself a package to a hotel where she will be staying. She travels with dried fruit, nuts, carrots, and apples.

Back home, she purchases organic foods through a local organic buying club. Every day, she eats at least twelve fruits and vegetables. "I make a salad, with sea greens, algae, things like that. I take a few supplements. Probiotics are critical." She doesn't eat meat or cheese and favors flax-seed-based and coconut oils. Her website is filled with daily advice like the value of mint and cilantro as cancer-fighting foods.

Fonfa's exercise regimen alternates days between a stationary bike and other activities. "I have a vibrating platform and I use hand weights. I have a hula hoop, a trampoline, a yoga mat, and I just alternate stuff. I'm not a runner. I don't want to do the same thing every day. When I wake up in the morning, I just do it. I do 20 minutes but you can do 10 minutes. The key is to choose something you will do. That keeps me going. I always take the stairs. If I am not carrying a heavy suitcase, I take the stairs."

Having been diagnosed after her last recurrence with stage 4 breast cancer, Fonfa believes her own life is testament to what she preaches. "I had 25 tumors on the left side. I'm still here. My health is excellent. I am living proof you can survive."

———◦《◦》◦———

Johanna Littleton, a reading recovery program specialist for the Meridian, Mississippi, public school system, discovered a lump in her chest in 2013, when she was gardening.

"I sat down in the yard on a bench and my son put his head on my chest. He said, 'oh, you have a lump in your chest,'" said Littleton, forty-four, who has been married nineteen years and has an eight-year-old son.

Previous mammograms "never picked it up. I called my doctor and I told the receptionist I needed a mammogram because I found a lump. She got me in the next day, which was a Friday."

By Monday, she had her results: stage 2, triple-negative breast cancer. By Wednesday, she had a lumpectomy on her right breast. Genetic testing found she had the BRCA2 mutation, raising her risk significantly of ovarian and breast cancer.

Because of the test results, her breast surgeon suggested she undergo a double mastectomy. She agreed. "He said the cancer could recur in the other breast or the ovaries." He also told her to see her gynecologist about a preventive hysterectomy. "I told him I already had a partial hysterectomy for fibroid tumors. He said, 'we need to take the other ovary as well.' So that's what I did."

Littleton leaned toward reconstruction at the time of her diagnosis. "I was kind of for having it, having some kind of boob there," she said. She changed her mind when she and her husband met with a plastic surgeon.

"They showed me pictures. I just wasn't happy in all honesty with the way they look. They were real Frankenboobie looking. They really were like Barbie Frankenstein. I honestly thought I'd rather have nothing because I'd seen the pictures of women with nothing online. And of course, they are all beautiful women with a beautiful new chest."

The more she thought about going flat, the more comfortable she got with the idea. "I honestly thought I'd rather be that kind of pretty than have Frankenboobies with no nipples. The surgeon was adamantly against doing the nipple sparing because the lump was right there. So I'd have those Barbie doll boobs with big scars across them and no sensation in my chest. It would be strictly for aesthetic reasons. They would be there to please everybody else when I wore clothes."

"We deliberated for weeks on this. It got to be where we could please everybody else or we could just be happy with me. And so we decided to go a little natural and let me be me. When we made that decision, that's when we talked to our son about it. We explained what I was going to have done. We looked at some pictures like the one of the lady on the beach in a bikini bottom. The most beautiful women. He was all for it."

In 2014, she had a double mastectomy and the rest of a total hysterectomy and oophorectomy. The day her husband helped her take the bandages off her chest, "I was extremely unhappy. I still had my drains in. I had an allergic reaction to the tape. I started to bleed under the tape."

She called her doctor's office to come in. "It took him a couple hours to unbandage my chest. That was the first time I saw it. I thought, oh my god, I screwed up. Give me Frankenboobs please. I'm serious."

Her husband's jokes assured her things would be fine. "He's always kind to boost up how pretty I am without any breasts," Littleton said.

She went to the Internet to find support. "I joined a couple of groups on Facebook to figure out how to cope. It's not that I was unhappy with what I lost. I was mourning the loss of my boobs. I didn't just lose my boobs, I lost my ovaries. I lost my womanhood. I came out of it feeling very, very de-womanized. I lost my hair and when it grew back, I lost the color in my hair. I'm grey now."

As she recovered from surgery, "when I put on comfortable clothes, because my skin is so sensitive where I had the surgery, I wear my husband's T-shirts, which are a double extra-large shirt. I look like an old man. My gut sticks out because I'm overweight. I'm heavy. I look like an old man with a beer gut. When I had boobs, you didn't notice the gut as much. I don't have that camouflage now."

"At first, I thought I had done myself an injustice. One day, my little boy came up and kissed me and said, 'you're so pretty mom.' I decided to say, screw it. It's about who you are. He wasn't seeing my boobs. So I went out and started taking advice from other people and I started looking at the clothes in my closet. I found clothes in cheap stores. We don't make much and we are supporting a big, extended family. So I went to places like T.J. Maxx. I found some diagonal-striped shirts and some big clunky necklaces. Things like that. I put them on and I said, 'hey, I may look flat-chested but I still look like a girl.' That made me feel a lot better about my decision."

Littleton had no interest in wearing a prosthesis. "I don't want the illusion of something being there when there is nothing there. If I wanted that, I should have had reconstruction. It gets back to the idea of, am I getting it to please everybody else or do I need to be happy with who I am? Everybody except for my brother and husband and my son wanted me to have reconstruction. It's the men in my life who accepted it. Doesn't that tell you something about society's expectations about body image?"

She wishes more doctors and breast cancer books were honest about recuperation issues and complications of mastectomy and breast reconstruction.

"No one really tells you about the worst part, which is the recuperation. I wasn't scared about losing my breast. I think I was prepared for it. But nobody tells you, this is how it is going to feel when you recuperate from it. They say, the worst part is behind you. Bullshit. That was the easy part."

"The worst part is at home. You are so swollen from the trauma to the tissue and the drains. There's all kinds of stuff that nobody ever talks about. Even the groups. They post about what clothing you can wear with the drains but not how you are going to feel. You feel miserable. I was in so much pain and I didn't know it was from the drains. When they pulled the drains from my right chest, it was an immediate relief. I looked down and said, 'God, I felt so much better.' I was not ready to run a marathon but I felt better. The doctor said, 'oh yes, the drains cause a lot of discomfort.' I said 'why didn't you guys tell me this?' Because when I'm lying in bed, moaning and groaning to my husband, and I am not sleeping well because I have this pain in my chest, not from where the stitches are because that area is numb, I wish people would be more honest and upfront about the actual recuperation. When you ask questions about recuperation, they say, 'just take it easy.' You get all these cliché phrases."

"The more blunt and honest the doctor is, the more prepared I can be," she added.

On her right side, where her breast surgeon did a more extensive mastectomy than on the left, Littleton developed lymphedema in her arm and on the side of her chest.

"It gets real bad in my chest actually," said Littleton. "I get it underneath my underarm. I have a lymphedema specialist I went to who showed me how to do exercises and showed me how to massage the swelling out." She wears a thick, "super ugly" compression vest at home for the pain and swelling.

"My lymphedema hurts the bicep in my arm, where you make a muscle, and under my underarm. It will swell so much it will look like I'm carrying a side boob."

She underwent ten weeks of therapy for the problem in 2015. Between the therapy and the vest, "the only pain I have, I get a muscle cramp like a charley horse where my right boob used to be. I get 'em once every two or three days. They last 5–15 minutes. I can be anywhere. I'll be eating in a restaurant or teaching in my classroom. I put my right thumb on the scar of the mastectomy and pull that muscle and stretch to the left. It will happen in the car when I put a seat belt on."

She planned to return later in the summer to see her doctor about the problem.

Her only regret, she said, was thinking that she'd end up with a pair of breasts like the ones she found on the Internet, when she looked for mastectomy photos on plastic surgery center websites.

She sure doesn't look like that, she said. "Your chest is not a smooth, flawless thing. It's extremely ugly to look at. You look up mastectomy pictures online, you always have these really smooth scars. My surgeon said, 'you will too. It takes time.' Well, it's been almost a year since my mastectomy. My scars are starting to smooth out. But is my chest pretty? No it is not. When I speak to other women, they say I should have plastic surgery on my chest."

"So even if you are flat and fabulous, you still have this pressure to go in to the plastic surgeon to smooth your chest out. I'm not lying to you. You've got the dog-ears, the lumps and the bumps. To this day, I get pressure to reconstruct. To this day, people tell me, it's not too late."

———— »«●»« ————

Sharon Fitzpatrick Blain, sixty-eight, of Grosse Pointe Farms, Michigan, met with a plastic surgeon after her 1999 breast cancer diagnosis but had more pressing issues to address than breast reconstruction.

She had a stage 2 invasive lobular breast tumor found on an annual mammogram, with three positive lymph nodes, requiring surgery, chemotherapy, and radiation.

Blain is a retired pediatric clinical nurse specialist, and, by her own description, a lifelong worrier. Her personality, and her son's pending high school graduation, led her to quickly feel comfortable with getting a bilateral mastectomy without construction.

"Reconstruction just wasn't important," she said. "The worrier in me was considering possible complications, if I developed an infection, if I didn't heal as I was supposed to. It would delay the chemo. There was no way I wanted to do that. I just wanted to heal. I had to wait a minimum of six weeks after my surgery before I could start the chemo. So I thought, that brings us up to graduation. I didn't want to interfere with that at all. So that's what went into the decision not to do any reconstruction. Maybe we'll think about this down the road."

Blain's specific tumor played a role in her decision, too. Lobular tumors have a higher chance of recurring. She knew a lumpectomy would mean monitoring herself for cancer for the rest of her life. "I had to recognize that this is who I am and I can't worry about it 24 hours a day. Is it showing up today? Am I going to need mammograms every three months? So I knew myself and I knew my limitations."

Fortunately, Blain and her husband were able to quickly find a good medical team through the Henry Ford Health System, in Detroit, Michigan. "We've been part of the Henry Ford Health System for thirty-five years. We knew that their cancer program was affiliated with the University of Michigan. We felt, we're not going to search somewhere else. I have one friend who has been all over the United States. She's had treatments in New York and Texas. She just goes everywhere. I don't feel that way. I felt very confident in what we had here was as good as it could be. That was another thing. Sandy and I established, between the two of us, confidence in our team. It really helped cement the feeling that we're in good hands."

Blain completed her first round of chemotherapy. Sure enough, "my hair all fell out the day of Peter's graduation" while she was showering to get ready to go. She walked into a computer room and said to her two sons, "OK guys, this is it. Here's the day we knew it would come." They said, "OK, Mom."

Frugal by nature, Blain "was ready with my scarf. I decided I wasn't going to wear a wig. I didn't want to spend money on something I hopefully wouldn't need in a year."

Her bilateral mastectomy was a same-day procedure.

Because of the surgical drains and dressings, she slept on her back, "and I had to be all propped up because your muscle has been cut and you have drains to empty. Sandy would help put me in bed and prop me up with pillows. It was a challenge. He'd have to lift me and help walk me to the bathroom."

"The first week was the tough one. After that, it was still awhile before I could get my chest wet. That was the other thing, when the drains had to be emptied and the bandages came off, I couldn't look at it. Sandy would have to inspect it for me. It took me awhile to look at it. I'd look up or I'd close my eyes."

"It was very emotional. I remember the night before surgery I looked in the mirror at myself. I thought, this is the last time I see these. It was very, very hard. You see yourself with this incision from here to here and you realize how vulnerable you are and mutilated. In a good way, I'm so grateful they could do this. But this is your body and trauma has happened to your body. So it took me a while to look."

"A couple weeks passed. Little by little, I was feeling better. I couldn't shower because I had drains and the incision. I'd sit on a little stool in the bathtub and Sandy could help me. I'd tilt my head back so he could wash my hair. We had that little routine. It made me feel better. I wasn't feeling sorry for myself. It wasn't that. It just was a scary, emotional time. I prayed it would all be OK. I never looked back; I never second-guessed about it. I thought, as I got healthier, should I get reconstruction?"

Blain appreciated her husband's help as well as understanding to give her the space she needed at times. "Sandy is not an emotional person. He was just there. He just kind of did things. He didn't hover. He was there when I needed him. He was very tender and caring. But he didn't go overboard pampering me. He didn't make a big deal about going off to chemo. Once we got into a routine, I gradually started to cook dinner. Things just kind of evolved."

For the rest of the summer and fall, she continued chemotherapy. Her strength returned, but she developed mental fogginess and other "chemo brain" side effects, which she found "unsettling." She attended a breast cancer support group, Sharing & Caring, at Beaumont Hospital, Royal Oak, Michigan, one of the oldest and most established ones of its kind in the Detroit area.

"That was very helpful. All these women, so many, had it and they were calling it chemo brain. I'm sure at some level that lasted two to three years. It was a long time. It wasn't a matter of completing your chemo and all of a sudden your brain feels clear. It wasn't a constant thing but you just didn't feel clear-headed."

One of six children, Blain asked her siblings, as well as her close friends, to respect her viewpoint about her surgery decisions and medical appointments. "I said I know how well intentioned you are. Don't send me articles from around the country about other places." She also told them, "'Please don't ask me questions. Let me tell you. I said, 'I'll share with you. Please don't ask me, when I go to an appointment, don't ask me my prognosis. You can ask me how I'm feeling but please don't ask me specifics about my progress or some of the specifics about what the doctor has to say.' Everyone was great."

"I'm a private person. We have to do things in our own personal way and it's just as legitimate. We all have a different way of coping."

When she resumed chemotherapy, Blain protected herself from getting sick by staying home initially. As a result, she never got sick or developed an infection. By fall she was able to resume her job at the time as a special educational resource room assistant in the Grosse Pointe public school system, working with children with special needs.

Sixteen years later, she still has some pain from her mastectomy. She has "a sensation of tightness across my chest" at times and "a little limitation in range-of-motion on the right," she said. "I can feel there's a tension there. I had axillary dissection on both sides. They took 14 lymph nodes. You know you've got some nerve damage."

She feels it in yoga. "If I'm on my back, stretching my arms out, I can't stretch my right arm easily. It takes me awhile. I have to work at it. I can't put it straight out but it's not a limitation." She never has had lymphedema, a swollen arm problem.

She returned to her breast and plastic surgeon a few times after her mastectomy because "for a couple of years, I had a couple of areas that didn't heal well. Eventually that all healed."

Usually, Blain, who has a small, slender frame, favors camisoles and shirts and sweaters. She doesn't use breast forms, just a padded bra for dressy dresses. "I went to a couple of fitters and never found anything successfully," she said of the breast forms. "And I was so comfortable going without. Why spend all this money if I just use them for a special occasion?"

Still, she added, "There isn't a day I'm not reminded of it, but very quickly, in the same thought process, I am grateful I am here. So I don't have any issues with it. And Sandy doesn't. He's never indicated in any way that it is off-putting. He's very tender. It all transpired the way I thought it would. It was pretty seamless. I'm a happy woman."

Blain said she shared her story so other women know "there doesn't have to be pressure to do reconstruction. It's an individual decision."

"Women need to have confidence in themselves to decide for themselves. We get so influenced by external pressures. We have to do what's in our best interest and for our family."

————))((())((————

Natalie Palmer, fifty-two, of West Simsbury, Connecticut, was diagnosed with stage 4 breast cancer in 2005.

She postponed surgery for nearly a year to complete chemotherapy, as well as radiation to her liver, where tests found a few spots of cancer.

She had a unilateral mastectomy without reconstruction in 2006 and underwent surgery to remove her ovaries in January 2007.

"I really did not want surgery at all," said Palmer, who publishes an online wellness magazine for women with breast and other cancers called The Pink Paper, http://www.thepinkpaper.com. "But I decided if they take the breast, my body could concentrate on healing."

Ever since her diagnosis, Palmer has pursued the healthiest lifestyle she could. She credits her spirituality and healthy habits to the fact that she has lived ten years with a diagnosis of stage 4 cancer.

"The last time I went in for a PET (positron emission therapy) scan was three-and-a-half years ago," she said. She hasn't seen a surgeon in ten years.

"I attribute my survival to both a medical and holistic approach," she said. "I changed my diet completely; I eliminated all meat and dairy. I did that because my partner is involved with a food company founded by Seventh-Day Adventists, and a healthy diet and vegetarianism is a big part of their religion, and thinking about what you put into your body. I really embraced that. You have to have a holistic approach. So you look at your spiritual well-being and your medical issues."

"Adding exercise, doing yoga, and meditation, I guess I became friends with myself again. I let go as much as I could, and I'm still in the process of doing that."

"By no means have I really evolved to where I'd like to be. I forgave myself for some things. You know we all hold on to stuff we shouldn't. I believe that's huge and I prayed a lot. I believe that the spiritual part of making peace with yourself is important. I made peace, and I felt healed, whether the healing involved never having cancer again or if the healing was going to be part of my journey again. Whether I get cancer again, I still feel healed. That won't change. I feel I've done my absolute best."

Palmer uses a prosthesis form outside her home. After "trying them all," she found a lightweight model, called the Anita Care Equitex Breast Prosthesis, which she likes a lot. It fits into the pocket of a bra. It costs about $230, and is widely available at mastectomy retail stores and on Internet sites and is covered by most health insurance.

Her advice to women facing surgery decisions is to take it slowly. "They try to push things through. The medical teams make it like one-size-fits-all. Slow down. You don't need to make a decision tomorrow. Make an informed decision as best as you can. Listen to yourself. It's a huge deal. It's not a little deal. It's trauma to your body. You are going under the knife. It's not a little deal."

"There is time. I just took off one breast when I had stage 4 cancer. It's been almost 10 years now. I'm still here. I think the scare and the fear, maybe it's a little better but I don't think it has changed that much. You are pushed by fear. This is a decision that is permanent. It's your decision and it's important that you have somebody there with you when you go to your appointments, to advocate for you and to listen."

"You can't live in fear."

———

Jill Conley, a young woman with stage 4 breast cancer, caught the attention of several million people after she posed for a video in a stunning, pink toile ball gown under the Eiffel Tower in Paris in 2013.

The video of Conley, thirty-one, a tall, leggy brunette, shown both gowned and bare-chested, went viral and launched Conley on a new platform to bring hope and a positive body image to women with breast cancer, regardless of their stage of disease and whether they had reconstruction or not.[1]

She is one-breasted, after reconstruction with silicone implants failed in one of her breasts damaged by radiation treatments, a common problem. By then, she was much too focused on staying alive to be bothered by having just one breast.

"I want people with or without cancer to feel beautiful and sexy," said Conley, a model for a high-fashion mastectomy line, AnaOno Intimates. She has been a speaker at national cancer meetings and been a guest on national TV talk shows.

She also has used her fame to start the nonprofit Jill's Wish Foundation, which gives small grants to financially struggling breast cancer patients.

Conley was uninsured when she was diagnosed with breast cancer. In June 2015, the nonprofit held its second annual "Rock What You Got 5K Fundraiser" in Louisville to raise money for the grants. "Our mission is to raise money to help families going through cancer with their finances," Conley said, in a May 2014 interview. "The burden of the bills just start adding up, especially if you can't work."

Initially, like many women, Conley said she felt disfigured after her surgery. "After my double mastectomy I just stared in the mirror for hours." Her huband, Bart , asked why she was upset. "I said, Bart, you'll never understand this. It's like if you had your penis cut off tomorrow. He said, 'No it's not, that's totally different.' I said, 'No, it's not.' From a young age, women have been exposed to magazine images and stuff like that; it's hard. They are your breasts."

"Every time I look in the mirror now, all I think of is, damn, I'm alive. These are war wounds and I went through a war and I'm standing here."

"I never look at my chest and oh my God, say it's disgusting. I have so much pride. I don't want to sound conceited. I look at my chest . . . to me it's like beautiful. I went through so much. So did my husband and family and I'm still here."

"Boobs are overrated."

Conley died February 2, 2016, of breast cancer. She was 38. Her YouTube video shows how she conveyed important messages about living with breast cancer.[1]

10

Uneven Results

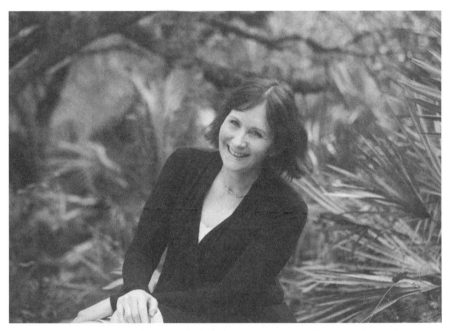

Betti Adams says her mismatched breasts are "a smallie, not a biggie."

Enough. At least for now. Perhaps forever.

Women with unfinished breast reconstruction have varying reasons for postponing or never completing the work.

Sometimes they've just had enough surgery, particularly if they developed problems before.

Some wait to give their bodies a break before going back.

Sometimes, they stop because the problems they develop seem unfixable, sometimes even to their own plastic surgeons.

And many say that after surviving a breast diagnosis, living with imperfect breasts pales in comparison. "It is a smallie, not a biggie," is the way Betti Adams, sixty, of Delray Beach, Florida, put it.

Living with uneven or unfinished results of breast reconstruction was a little-discussed topic of conversation until recently. Now, it's a popular topic of discussion on Internet breast cancer support group message boards, where women share their views about a wide range of topics, including leaving well enough alone, once they had had one breast reconstruction procedure that did not live up to their expectations.

What causes one woman to return for what may be multiple revision surgeries while another may say, no thanks, that's enough?

The Michigan Breast Reconstruction Outcome Study, one of the few patient satisfaction studies on the issue, found that women weren't as happy if they developed a complication from breast reconstruction, were older, or had reconstruction with implants.[1]

A strong predictor of the unhappiness was the development of a complication that involved either breast implants or a choice to preventively remove a second noncancerous breast, the study found.

These stories shared by Betti Adams, Maria Cruz Castellanos, and Rose Gow help explain some of the broader reasons why some women live with what they've got.

————— ◄(0)► —————

With a family history of ovarian and breast cancer, Betti Adams, an Internet consultant who works from her home, knew she should have been more regular about checking her breasts for lumps.

"I actually did not regularly do breast self-exams," Adams said. "I am not very organized or scheduled. I'm more the type to do it when I heard of someone being diagnosed or after seeing a public service announcement, then forgetting it for the rest of the year. I always felt a twinge of guilt when my gynecologist or mammogram technician would say, 'You do monthly self-exams, don't you?' I feel this is an important part of my story since I might have found it much sooner and it would have been smaller if I had done monthly self-exams."

A sore on her nipple made her examine her breast more closely, and she found a lump, she said.

Lodged behind her nipple, the lump had not turned up on Adams's last mammogram. Her doctor agreed to follow it closely.

A second mammogram confirmed she had a breast tumor that had spread aggressively, requiring chemotherapy and radiation. She had a double mastectomy with saline implant reconstruction in 2004. At the time, a federal moratorium on silicone implants, lifted two years later, limited most women to saline implants. Adams said, "I read so much negative about silicone I chose saline."

Thin, tall, and small-breasted, Adams said she was told she didn't have enough tummy fat for a tissue-transfer procedure. That left saline implants. She found the process of expanding her chest skin to hold a permanent implant uncomfortable, as do many women. It was an ordeal but she got through it, she said.

She was happy to exchange the temporary saline expanders for permanent ones, which she has to this day.

"Do I want more surgery? Not really. The nurse practitioner at my oncologist's office said it looks like one of them might be a little encapsulated," or hardened, she said. "I asked her, 'is that bad?' and she said, not if it doesn't bother you."

Adams describes the shape of her reconstructed breasts at various times as "weird, small and moundlike." They give her no sensation. "I think they are ugly. It's not something you show off."

The new look surprised her a little at first. "After you have a mastectomy, the big surprise for me was not realizing that the breasts I got would not be anything like real breasts," she said. "If the benefit of having cancer is that you get a great new pair or better than the ones you had before, then we're not there yet," she said, laughing at references many people make about the positive benefits for women about breast reconstruction.

Adams does not have nipples or areola, like many women with unfinished reconstruction. Her plastic surgeon discouraged her from completing that part, she said. No problem. "I don't miss them much," she said of her nipples.

"My husband and I talked about it and we talked about it with the plastic surgeon. He wasn't really encouraging. The doctor said of nipple reconstruction, 'They're OK in the best cases,'" Adams said, recalling what the doctor told her. "He said it hasn't really been perfected to the point where people are thrilled with them."

Adams favors camisoles and blouses but dresses up for events at her local synagogue, where she is active. "I already had my children," said Adams, who has two grown daughters and a stepson. "I used my breasts for what God intended. I think people and bodies adjust amazingly to whatever comes their way."

Adams uses her story to tell her two daughters that "looks aren't really that important. Things change. I've learned to live with it."

Fortunately for her, her husband is loving and accepting of her new body, Adams said.

"I thought this was the sweetest thing," she said. "I had said to him, 'look at me, I don't feel pretty.' He said, 'I would love you if you were a piece of bread lying on the ground.'"

———⊃●(❀)●⊂———

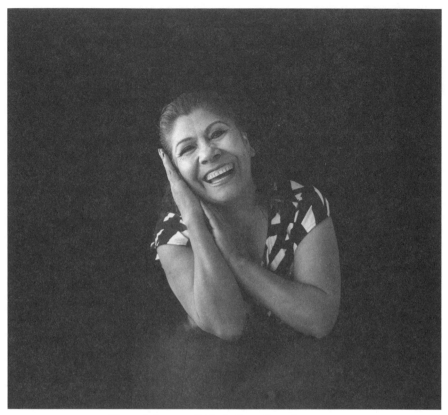

"Enough for now," Maria Cruz Castellanos says.

Surgery complications have kept Maria Cruz Castellanos, fifty-five, of Summit, Illinois, from returning to finish her breast reconstruction.

During a unilateral reconstruction procedure in 2006, using tissue, fat, and blood vessels from her back and butt to make a new breast, she had a rare complication and went into respiratory shock. Chemotherapy for her aggressive cancer before the surgery also weighed on her.

She had a tough recovery for several months. She plunged into depression, making her doubt her decision to even have breast reconstruction.

"I got severely depressed," she said. "I cried a lot constantly. At that time I didn't know much about breast cancer. I asked myself, 'Why me, why not someone else?' The truth is that if I had known more about cancer, I would not have done it. Now that I know more, I think I would not have had the surgery."

She realizes she had breast reconstruction because she feared it would ruin her marriage if she didn't. "I thought, what if he leaves me? That is the reason sometimes you make the wrong decisions. You think about others and not yourself."

She also harbored irrational fears that more surgery would cause her cancer to return.

"I got scared," said Castellanos, a mother of four grown children. "I heard comments from people that the cancer will return. So much sacrifice and work and then for the cancer to return. I didn't want to do it because I feared it would come back. So I said, no more. This is enough. I don't want to go through this anymore."

Still, nine years later, she is considering going back to finish reconstruction.

Her breasts don't match, and one has no nipple or areola.

Castellanos volunteers as a patient advocate at a chemotherapy clinic at St. Anthony's Hospital, in Chicago, Illinois, where she helps out, including giving advice to women to get breast exams and to "keep going and be strong." With time, she has put the reasons for her depression into perspective.

"I look at other people going through tough times and they get through it. I asked myself, why can't I? You have to fight for your life. If God keeps us here it's because of a grand plan, a grand purpose, to be of service."

———◦《◍》◦———

Rose Gow, fifty-seven, a high school career development counselor from Macomb, Michigan, lives with two breasts reconstructed differently that don't match. She's had several dozen procedures and still is not done. Her plastic surgeon has told her he may not be able to help her any further.

Gow was diagnosed with breast cancer in 2008 after a routine mammogram at age fifty found she had an aggressive, triple-negative tumor. She had a lumpectomy and radiation. She wanted genetic testing but didn't get it because she couldn't afford the test and her and husband's health insurance policy would not pay for it at the time. In May 2015, the Obama administration ordered all health insurers to pay for all genetic testing and counseling "without cosharing" for those with a family history of breast or ovarian cancer, according to a May 11, 2015, story by health reporter Robert Pear.

Six months later, her sister, Eileen Kastura, was diagnosed with breast cancer, and Gow and her two sisters had genetic testing, which found they all had a BRCA mutation. The finding led to Gow's decision to return for a double mastectomy. "I talked about it, thought about it, researched it," said Gow, a mother with four grown children. "I decided that since I was so high risk, I didn't want to worry about living my life with MRIs and follow-up exams."

Gow had to wait nearly a year to have a double mastectomy because radiation treatment had caused extensive damage in her left breast, she said. Her plastic surgeon blamed radiation for her healing issues, she said. "I was going in every other week just to have the necrotic tissue taken off," she recalled. "All you had to do was push on the breast and there would be gushes of water."

She consider the problems might have been avoidable if she had had a double mastectomy, which she would have chosen if she knew she had the gene mutation. "Had I had the testing, I would have had a double mastectomy. I wouldn't have gone through that." The failure of her health coverage to pay for genetic testing at the time also riles her because if she had been tested and found out she carried the BRCA gene, her sister likely would have been diagnosed earlier with breast cancer, at an earlier stage, she said.

"It makes me angry," she said. "I would have had a better outcome. My sister probably would have found out she had breast cancer earlier than she did. I don't know if her outcome would have been different if they had caught it at an earlier stage than stage 3. She went in immediately to test herself after I was diagnosed. I didn't have $4,000 to $5,000 to pay for it. Being I was the first in the family to get it, I didn't expect that I had the gene. Most definitely all this plays into what I think and still do."

After she healed, Gow's plastic surgeon performed breast reconstruction with silicone implants, but she developed one problem after another during the temporary expander phase. "We were trying to do expanders and implants on both sides but I had problems with necrosis," or deadening of the skin. "There were multiple times I had to have skin taken away. It was quite grueling. I had probably, all in all, twenty surgeries related to the expanders."

Concluding that her left breast was too thin and weakened by radiation damage to support a breast implant, the surgeon reconstructed her left breast with an abdominal tissue-transfer procedure and her healthy right breast with a silicone implant.

Seven years and extra pounds later, Gow has lopsided breasts without nipples or areola.

A back problem and cancer treatments caused her to gain weight only in the breast reconstructed with her tissue, not the implanted one. "Although a breast and nipples don't define you, I don't look normal," she said. "I don't feel normal." She also lives with chronic pain. "I have a lot of numbness if I move a certain way because I have no abdominal muscle. I get a lot of cramping on my left side. It doesn't happen all the time. If I'm standing up in the shower or bend down to wash my legs, I'll get that cramp. I have to get it together and do deep breathing to get rid of it."

The problems made her depressed and adversely affected her marriage, she said. "We really need to start looking at when women start going through these things, that before they go through them, there really needs to be a plan in place where the couples go to counseling. The husband needs to know what is going to happen and how their wife is going to look and how she's going to heal because it's hard for us to say this. We're already dealing with emotions. They have no idea how you'll look and feel so different."

Gow likes her reconstructed breast made with a silicone implant. "The right side looks great," she said. "It looks like a real breast. The left side is misshapen. It's very tight. I don't have a shelf. I can't wear a bra because if I do, it just rolls right up around my neck. There's nothing to hold it. There's nothing really I can do about it. There are some clothes I can't wear because of it."

She has kept in touch with her plastic surgeon, but "he has not seemed receptive to trying to make things work a little bit more," she said. "I think he feels he's reached the maximum of what he can do. It may be he can't go any further." She wonders, though. "I watched that TV program *Botched*. They actually can go in and help people."

Her plan for now is to lose weight, eat healthier, exercise more, and continue therapy about living with chronic pain. With time, Gow said she's learned to live with her less-than-perfect breasts.

"Living with it is just something you have to learn to adapt to. There are other people who have limbs cut off, something you need to walk with or to hug your children or your family. Losing a limb is probably worse than losing a breast."

And yes, despite all the surgeries, "I probably would do it over again, just because of my age. I don't think I would have wanted to live life without breasts."

11

Delayed Reconstruction

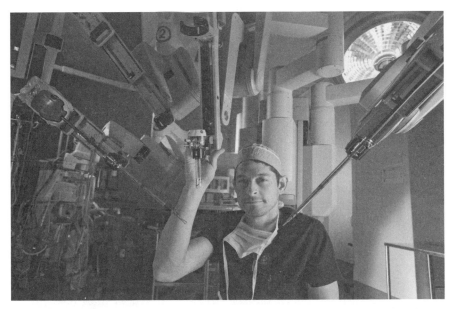

Dr. Jesse Selber has developed a minimally invasive robotic technique to perform breast reconstruction. Photo courtesy of Dr. Jesse Selber.

Attention to breast reconstruction advances has obscured one long-time reality: most American women don't have reconstruction. The ones that do may wait.

In 2014, 102,200 women underwent breast reconstruction. Data from the American Society of Plastic Surgeons show that 71,326 reconstruction procedures were done immediately at the time of mastectomy and 30,889 were delayed.[1]

Some women need time to sort out their options and give their bodies time to heal. And increasingly, women wait because they have larger or more problematic tumors that call for chemotherapy or radiation.

The use of these therapies, delivered before and after surgery, motivated doctors to rethink the best timing for reconstruction in women having radiation as part of their treatment.

There's still no consensus about the best time to do reconstruction in these patients, and women are likely to get conflicting opinions from different doctors.

"In cases where radiation is planned following mastectomy, immediate reconstruction remains controversial," said Dr. Edwin Wilkins, professor of plastic surgery at the University of Michigan, Ann Arbor. "I think it's safe to say that most surgeons still prefer to delay reconstruction until radiation has been completed."

Still, some doctors perform reconstruction at the time of mastectomy "with full knowledge that the reconstruction will be radiated," he said.

Doctors use both implant and tissue reconstruction after radiation, but "there is some evidence that abdominal flap reconstruction procedures may tolerate radiation better than implants," Wilkins said.

In implant reconstruction, doctors also disagree about whether radiation should be done after temporary expanders are put in place or whether radiation should wait until the complete implant exchange is done with permanent implants, he said. "Clearly, we need better evidence to answer these questions," Wilkins said.

Dr. Steven Kronowitz, professor of plastic surgery at the University of Texas MD Anderson Cancer Center in Houston, Texas, developed what he calls "delayed immediate reconstruction" in 2002 as one option, now adopted by other top centers.

In delayed immediate reconstruction, doctors place a temporary saline implant into the chest when performing a mastectomy. The adjustable device, the mainstay of implant reconstruction, stretches the skin to eventually hold a permanent implant while doctors wait for pathology results from sentinel or lymph node biopsies to determine if a tumor has spread.

The filling procedure continues in women whose tumors have not spread to the tested lymph nodes. If cancer is found, doctors deflate the implant temporarily and begin radiation.

After radiation is done, the implant is usually traded for a permanent silicone device. The use of acellular dermal matrix (ADM) products made from sterilized human and animal collagen products add additional support and contour to breasts thinned or damaged by radiation.

Kronowitz said women who delay immediate reconstruction have fewer complication rates with reconstruction after radiation. Many are grateful to be eligible for reconstruction, he said.

The MD Anderson program considers radiation planning, and the precision of it to be so important that it brings in radiation oncologists for presurgery evaluations of patients, Kronowitz said. "It's evolved to when the patient needs radiation they come to our clinic and our physician assistant will look at how the chest geometry looks. They get a computerized tomography or CT scan before radiation. That's how they design and position their radiation beams to minimize the impact on the heart and lungs."

Coupled with nipple-sparing mastectomy approaches, "this really is changing the tide," said Dr. Jesse Selber, a microvascular plastic surgeon on the MD Anderson team. He is developing a robotic approach to make breast reconstruction minimally invasive. He has performed about fifty of the procedures since he began doing them five years ago at MD Anderson. It is the only robotic plastic surgery program in the world for breast reconstruction, he said. It can be done with either implants or a woman's own tissue.

In robotic breast reconstruction, Selber makes a small incision in the armpit to either place an implant or obtain a flap of tissue from the back known as the latissimus dorsi muscle. "The significance is, we can perform the procedure with only a small incision in the armpit," Selber said. "Back incisions don't tend to heal very well. So it can be slightly uncomfortable with a pretty long incision" from conventional back flap procedures, he said.

Women eligible for the surgery "are a pretty select group," he said. "It's for women who are a little thin and aren't candidates for an abdominal flap, but would benefit from autologous tissue," he said. "If they'd had decent good expansion of the skin but for whatever of a variety of reasons such as radiation they need protection between the implant and the skin, this is a nice option that makes use of the latissimus muscle without the undesirable back incision that usually accompanies it."

Selber added, "We have an entire set of clinical algorithms and approaches, based on the size of the breast and where the lump that has to be removed is located that we use," he said. "They mostly follow patterns of breast reduction concepts. So we look at a lumpectomy essentially as a reduction, but we don't get to choose the part that gets reduced. The robotic latissimus harvest fits into this algorithm for reconstruction of upper outer quadrant lumpectomies."

He is teaching others and expects the program to grow. "We do about two of these a month. We'll probably do more as we go on. I'm starting to teach others."

Kimberlee Mitchell, fifty, of Decatur, Alabama, one of Selber's robotic patients, is very happy with her delayed robotic reconstruction with silicone implants. "Robotics absolutely gave me a sense of normalcy," said Mitchell, who is married and has two sons, seventeen and twelve. The oldest is a special needs child, and his and the family's schedule, plus her job as executive director of the Carnegie Visual Arts Center in Decatur, influenced her choice of surgery. "This was a good alternative for me, given what I wanted my life to be like after this was over," she said.

Mitchell said she only has a couple of faint scars from the robotic procedure. Mitchell outright rejected reconstruction with her own tissue as
disfiguring. "The scarring has been really minimal. Most of my scars are
from my mastectomy, not my robotic surgery. I just have three little scars,
on the side next to my rib cage. You really have to look for them. I was
wearing a bikini after I had my surgery. I am very happy with them. It has
enabled me to be active again and feel strong. You can take care of your
family. It's not the end. You can still go on and feel productive. It's not a
cakewalk. But you can still feel good about yourself and feel productive.
I don't have to stop and think about cancer every single day of my life. I
can go on and accomplish what I wanted to accomplish before cancer got
in the way."

Mitchell said she was quickly able to get to work and her routines. "I
work out with a personal trainer. I lift weights. I run. I like to be active. I
kayak, canoe and camp. I do boy-mom things like soccer and play football
in the yard. There's nothing I can't do."

––––––––«(●)»––––––––

Doctors have come to near agreement that overall, tissue-based reconstruction is more successful than reconstruction with implants, Kronowitz and Wilkins said.

"I think there's a fairly wide consensus that if you are doing delayed
reconstruction and a patient already has had a mastectomy and radiation,
tissue flaps do better," Wilkins said.

Kronowitz agreed. "Radiation and implants don't go together very
well. A large number of patients will form a contracture, a hard scar,
around the implant. It's the body's mechanism of walling off the body
from a foreign body. There's probably some genetic makeup that de-
termines whether people get thick scars or thin scars. And certainly
we know that radiation has a big impact on the inflammatory process.
There's a tendency towards not only loss of the implant but also capsular
contracture which can happen over time and be painful and lead to significant deformity."

"Complications are about four times higher in patients who got radiation. The numbers vary from implant loss of less than 10% to over 50%.
It just depends on the study. But invariably, with radiation, autologous
tissue tends to fare better," though many women aren't eligible because
they are too thin or too heavy, he said.

Women also may have to find out about tissue reconstruction on their
own. It may not be the first choice they hear about.

––––––––«(●)»––––––––

When Suzanne Simon, seventy-three, of West Bloomfield, Michigan, a retired preschool teacher, heard that her results might be better with tissue reconstruction, she bravely changed her mind.

At the time, she was in the expander phase of silicone breast reconstruction.

Just a few months before, in December 2011, Simon found a lump in her breast while turning over in bed. She wanted to get the issue resolved quickly because she is a busy woman who was leaving soon for a family wedding in California. She and her husband, married twenty-five years, have four grown daughters. She is a long-time board member and past president of the National Council of Jewish Women, Greater Detroit section.

Simon returned from the wedding with a call from her doctor as she got off the plane, telling her she had breast cancer.

She found a team at Beaumont Hospital in Royal Oak, Michigan, she respects and liked a lot, but she also made an appointment for a second opinion at the University of Michigan.

"U-M wanted to do surgery right away. Beaumont said do the oncology first, it will shrink the tumor." She had a stage 2 tumor and she would need surgery, chemotherapy, and radiation.

After asking around and doing research, finding that some leading centers prefer adjuvant therapy to begin prior to surgery, she opted for chemotherapy first.

Chemotherapy stretched from February to May, followed by a lumpectomy in June, a mastectomy in July, and radiation in August and September. The radiation made her itchy, and she developed shingles, a possible complication.

She hoped the treatments would shrink her tumor and allow her to only need the lumpectomy. But Beaumont's tumor board, a group of specialists reviewing her case, thought in the end mastectomy was her best insurance against a recurrence.

She chose silicone implant reconstruction and was several weeks into the process when she saw her breast surgeon, Dr. Nayana Dekhne, on a return appointment.

She told Simon that the hospital had just recruited a new microvascular surgeon, Dr. Kongrit Chaiyasate, who specializes in tissue-based reconstruction, along with complex facial reconstruction cases. "With radiated skin like yours, this may be a better solution," Simon said her breast surgeon told her. "You might want to meet with him and decide what to do."

Simon had talked to her original plastic surgeon as well. He told her that reconstruction results with implants "were iffy" because she had prior radiation, she said. He offered to do a latissimus dorsi tissue–based procedure using a flap of tissue, blood vessels, and muscles from her back.

Simon met with Chaiyasate, who offered her a DIEP flap procedure. Because the DIEP flap does not take attached muscle, it seemed like a better choice to her, she said. "If I had not had that meeting with my breast surgeon, I would have had a latissimus dorsi flap," Simon said.

Chaiyasate said autologous procedures are best in women with prior radiation. "I would advise women who are going through radiation to consider the autologous reconstruction as I replace the unhealthy tissue that is left behind from radiation with healthy tissue from their own bodies," he said.

Simon found recovery from her DIEP flap procedure "a little uncomfortable," but she was in less pain compared to what she experienced after her mastectomy, she said. She spent five days in the hospital. She has a big hip-to-hip scar, but she said, "It doesn't bother me because it was worth it. It was a positive thing to bring my life back to normal."

Looking back, she is glad she changed her mind. "This was just to get back control over my life and having it be the way I wanted it to be. Some of my friends said, 'I'm surprised, Sue, you didn't seem like the kind of person to do reconstruction.'"

She tells them, "I just wanted to get dressed each day without thinking about breast cancer."

"I live my life the same as I did when I was 40 just with more aches and pains. I am still doing the same things I did then and I'm just as active. I know I'm 73 but I don't spend much time complaining about aches and pains."

After chemotherapy she lost thirty pounds. She likes how she looks. "Actually when I was diagnosed one of my daughters said to me, 'you are going to have bigger boobs mom.' I do. I'm perfectly happy with them and what they look like."

———————◦◦⟨⟨◎⟩⟩◦◦———————

Terri Coutee, fifty-nine, of Tucson, Arizona, took time to thoroughly investigate her options after a mammogram found that her breast cancer recurred in April 2014. Originally, in January 2002, she had two lumpectomies, chemotherapy, and radiation for a stage 1 tumor she found while examining herself.

Her breast surgeon suggested a magnetic imaging resonance (MRI) test, which found that she had two different types of cancer in her breasts, which is not uncommon. Her breast surgeon, Dr. Michele Ley, associate professor of surgery at the University of the Arizona Cancer Center, told her about her options and mentioned tissue-based reconstruction.

"The day she told me about these flaps, it just kind of clicked with me," said Coutee, who has been married thirty-seven years and is a mother with two grown sons. She is a long-time teacher of English as a second language.

"I totally respect everyone is different but I didn't want anything foreign in my body. The fact I could be my own tissue donor sparked my interest. That's the conversation that should be happening in a doctor's office. Women shouldn't just be told you need a mastectomy. They should be told you need a mastectomy but let's also talk about your options for reconstruction."

Coutee wore a prosthesis for seven months. "Initially I was happy to have clothing to look more natural. But I became very tired of them. They became heavy; they were hot to me. We took a couple of trips on an airplane and they moved around and did weird things."

She had to delay her decision while researching her options because she had two different cancer tests that came up with slightly different recommendations on whether she needed chemotherapy. Her medical oncologist recommended chemotherapy, which she strongly did not want to do.

"My husband is an engineer. We sat down, crunched numbers, looked at charts. We were ready for that appointment with the medical oncologist, who said, 'You know Terri, you are the perfect person to make this choice on your own because you've been through this before'."

By late November, she made her mind up about chemotherapy. "I chose not to do it," she said.

She and her husband scheduled a flight to San Antonio to meet with Dr. Minas Chrysopoulo with the PRMA plastic surgery group. She had reviewed Chrysopoulo's blog posts on his group's website about delayed procedures for radiated patients like her and hoped he would find her a candidate. He did. "When we left his office, it was the first sense of hope that my husband and I had had all year," she said. "We felt such a burden was lifted off our shoulders."

On December 1, 2014, she had breast reconstruction with a DIEP flap. Chrysopoulo told Coutee he had to remove a lot of scar tissue in her left breast and had to take out a larger flap of tissue as a result. "That's his skill. That breast is softer and I have greater range of motion than I've had in 13 years," she said.

The experience motivated Coutee to begin a blog, http://diepcjourney .com, in which she writes about a range of reconstruction issues, including recovery from surgery and traveling to other cities for reconstruction. She manages a closed Facebook group, www.facebook.com/groups/diepc journey, that provides information as well as a forum for women with questions about reconstruction. She also lobbied for passage of H.R. 2540, the Breast Cancer Patient Education Act.[2] The bill requires doctors to educate all women about their options after mastectomy, from breast forms to reconstruction.

Coutee returned to San Antonio in April 2015 for a fat-transfer procedure to move fat from her thighs to her breasts. She loves her breasts. "I
tell people they're mine, they're warm and they wiggle. And I think they
are fabulous."

————•《◉》•————

It took Diane Mapes nearly four years of chemotherapy, radiation,
multiple surgeries, and the use of an external tissue-stretching device to
get her breasts back.

She doesn't regret it.

In February 2011, she noticed an odd spot, what she called a tuck, on
her left breast under the nipple. A mammogram didn't detect anything.
An ultrasound, however, identified three masses, two in her left breast
and one in her right. A biopsy confirmed she had a stage 3 lobular tumor
in her left breast and a stage 2 lobular tumor in her right. She needed a
double mastectomy, chemotherapy, and radiation, or what Mapes calls
"the full Monty."

As a health writer at the Fred Hutchinson Cancer Research Center in
Seattle, Mapes, fifty-six, uses her talent to reeducate other women about
reconstruction issues. Her blog, http://doublewhammied.com, has carried essays about surgery, body image, and dating issues as a long-time
single woman.

Mapes talked to several doctors who told her that breast reconstruction
with implants was not an option because she had radiation damage to her
breast. She had no interest in tissue reconstruction because "I didn't want
my body carved up like a Thanksgiving turkey" and she did not want to
have a procedure that might take muscle from her abdomen or back. A
single woman, she also worried she would be "out of commission for a
lot longer" with autologous reconstruction.

The opinions sent her off on a fact-finding mission to find some other
way to "get her girls back," as she likes to say.

It led her to Brava,[3] an external tissue expander used for reconstruction
and nonsurgical breast enlargement.

Brava looks like a supersized bra in a futuristic action film. Its website
describes how it works, at http://brava.com. It has two parts: two semi-
rigid domes rimmed with silicone gel and a minicomputer component
that regulates tension within the domes. Brava must be worn ten hours a
day for about two to three weeks before fat-grafting surgery. The device
applies a pull on the chest wall to create a pocket for the fat.

In 1999, the federal Food and Drug Administration allowed the device
to be sold in the United States. It is available through some two hundred
physicians authorized by the company to use the device.

"As a writer, I went into research and information-gathering mode," Mapes said. She interviewed Dr. Roger Khouri, the Miami, Florida, plastic surgeon who invented the device, as well as several patients who used the device for reconstruction after breast cancer.

It sounded a little bizarre, but Mapes, who took up boxing after cancer treatment, decided she could handle it. "Women who go through breast cancer endure a lot," she said. "They're tough. We go through some pretty heavy-duty stuff."

The Brava device was uncomfortable, cut into her armpits, and caused her sleepless nights. But she got through it, and after about three weeks she went in for a fat-transfer procedure. Her plastic surgeon used a liposuction tool to remove fat from her thighs.

There were complications. The liposuction was painful and caused seromas, pockets of fluid, to build on both of her thighs. Mapes lost the nipple on her left side, a common occurrence with radiated tissue.

Undaunted, she returned to the Brava device and fat grafting. This time, she developed an infection in her right breast after the fat-transfer procedure, requiring her to be hospitalized for several days. She nursed herself back to good health and realized that rebuilding her breasts through fat grafting alone was too time consuming and arduous, she said. She talked to her plastic surgeon, who agreed she had enough new healthy fat in her breasts to try implant reconstruction. In the spring of 2014, she had saline tissue expanders put in, which were swapped for silicone in September 2014.

She said of her choice: "Implants I wouldn't have picked them. But you do what you have to do. I wanted to fill out my clothes again. I wanted to look in the mirror and not immediately see cancer. It was hard for me. I was really determined to get my girls back."

She doesn't know quite what to make of her new breasts.

"I call them the strangers beside me. They are foreign. They feel foreign. I haven't gotten to the point where I feel comfortable. I still have body discomfort. Also I have discomfort looking in the mirror. They kind of, sort of look like what I used to have. I'm trying hard not to be rejecting of them. I don't know if I like them or not," she said late in 2014.

By July 2015, Mapes's reconstruction was done. "I've had two sets of tattoos early this year, which made a big difference with regard to how I felt about the 'new girls,'" she said in an email asking for an update. "Once I got my tattoos they finally looked more like actual boobs when I glanced in the mirror. That was great. But the new girls are nothing like the old girls. Reconstructed breasts are not the same as your old breasts and never will be and that's been a hard lesson for me to learn. At the back of your mind, you keep thinking you're going to get back the pieces of yourself that you lost to cancer. But you don't. You basically get boobs that look like boobs (implants) or boobs that feel like boobs (flap) but you don't get both."

"I'm still trying to figure out how much imperfection I can live with, and how much pain. I feel as if I have cereal bowls on my chest a lot of the time, even though I have a lot more fat than most people who've had reconstruction with implants. Physical therapy helped me stretch out the muscle so I don't have as much pain as I did earlier on but the implants always feel like I'm wearing the world's most uncomfortable bra, even when I'm not wearing a bra."

"I hate to sound so discouraging about reconstruction. It was extremely important for me to get my own back and I'm glad I went through it but it hasn't been easy. I miss my girls. I miss my nipples. I miss having sensation. And I'm not too hip to having fake boobs and all the new scars on my body, including the cannula scars from micro fat grafting. But hey, I can wear bras and shirts and no longer feel self-conscious about my chest. And I'm alive, so there's that."

12

The Nipple: The Ultimate Challenge

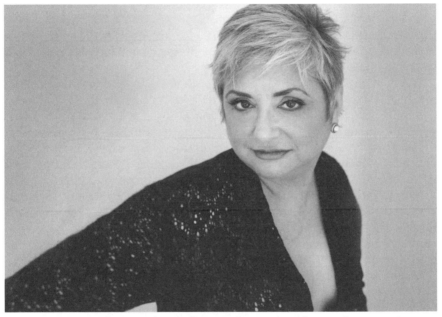

Donna Dauphinais took a ten-hour road trip to have her nipples tattooed.

Donna Dauphinais and her mother, Dorothy, packed overnight bags for a ten-hour drive east from their Grosse Pointe, Michigan, homes for Donna's appointment the next day to get her nipples tattooed by acclaimed breast cancer tattoo artist Vinnie Myers.

Dauphinais, fifty-five, an academic consultant, was in the final stages of getting new breasts after a double mastectomy in September 2011.

Now, more than two years later, she needed what Myers calls the cherries on the cupcake.

Since 2002, Myers, who has a sister who is a breast cancer survivor, has exclusively made nipple and areola tattoos for more than five thousand women, both those with breast cancer and others who undergo double mastectomies to prevent them from getting it. His clientele come from all over the country to his studio, Little Vinnie's Tattoos in Finksburg, Maryland, an hour's drive north of Baltimore.

With business growing as his fame spreads, Myers has added a second breast tattoo artist. He also sees women every month at the Center for Restorative Breast Surgery, a leading New Orleans plastic surgery center.

Myers charges $600 for a single-sided nipple and areola tattoo and $800 for both sides, up from the $600 Dauphinais paid the year before for bilateral tats. He creates conventional tattoos as well new 3-D types that give the illusion of a nipple or areola.

One in five is a redo for women who don't like the nipple tattoos they got elsewhere. He sees women whose nipples don't match, are barely visible, or "stick out like Vienna sausages," Myers said. "The areola can be painted too big, like a bull's-eye. The pigments used in medical offices often fade over a few years."

"Ours don't fade," he said. "We don't like redos. And we don't charge for them. We pride ourselves getting it right the first time."

Nipples may be the breast's crowning glory, but they are often a surgical afterthought. Usually, they are made from tissue from underarm breast surgery scars, eyelids, the inner thigh, and even the butt, then spliced together like a cord. Doctors tuck them into areas by folding back a flap of tissue along a mastectomy scar to add the newly created nipple.

Nipple construction can be done at the time of a mastectomy, as insurance may require, or later, in an outpatient procedure. Some women add nipples one side at a time. And in another separate procedure, the areolas are inked in and the nipples are darkened or lightened, usually by nurses at plastic surgery centers.

Myers is highly critical of the tattoos done in medical office settings. "I've never seen one that is good," he said. "Never." He's equally appalled that many breast cancer surgeons never talk to their patients about the reconstruction process, he said. "Something has to change with that because they are millions of women walking around with poor tattoos or no tattoos because of it," said Myers, who helped to create the Pink Ink Project, http://www.pinkinkproject.com, a website to help women find breast tattoo artists.

Myers also coauthored a report in the May 2014 issue of *Plastic and Reconstructive Surgery* describing what he and several prominent plastic surgeons called "superior aesthetic outcomes" with three-dimensional nipple and areola tattoos.[1] Dr. Eric Havorson, a Boston plastic surgeon at Brigham & Women's Hospital and lead author of the report, said he no longer does breast tattoo work "because of the outstanding results achieved by professional artists."

"Basic fundamentals of tattooing have also been ignored in traditional nipple-areola complex tattoo (e.g., machine speed, needle type, and color mixing)," the report said. "Medical practitioners often use preset speeds in excess of 180 cycles per second. This is twice the frequency of traditional tattooing and typically involves thin or compromised skin. The result is increased healing time, scarring, and poor pigment retention. It is not uncommon for patients to require two sessions for adequate pigmentation."

Ink used in doctors' offices for tattoos "are typically vegetable oil–based dyes or metal salt pigments mixed very thin and available in a small range of colors, limiting the choices available," the report said. "It is widely known that medical tattoos fade with time, sometimes becoming invisible after several years. By using traditional tattoo pigments and a color wheel, excellent color match can be achieved with significantly improved pigment retention."

The report added that "while referring patients to tattoo artists for 3-D nipple and areola construction may take some business away from a surgeon's practice, it is our obligation to offer patients the best results possible."

Web and medical industry savvy, Dauphinais did her research throughout her breast cancer treatment to familiarize herself with the issues she faced. Just by entering two words—nipple reconstruction—on Internet search engines, she found enough negative stories to worry her, including nipples that collapse or look overly small, like hers, or areolar tattoos that fade in a few years.

With insurance to cover her reconstruction—guaranteed by federal law for women after a mastectomy—Dauphinais booked an October 2013 appointment with Myers, whose studio in a nondescript strip mall is frequented by thousands of women who have flown or driven in for tattoos.

The morning of Dauphinais's appointment, two other women had flown into Baltimore from Ann Arbor, Michigan, and Boston, Massachusetts, to see Little Vinnie, who actually is a tall, lean guy in a porkpie hat, tie, vest, shirt, and jeans. Dauphinais had waited more than eighteen months for her new nipples.

Her reconstruction was delayed while she healed from recurrent infections in one of her breasts, requiring the removal of a temporary implant or expander used to stretch the chest wall before a doctor could put in a silicone implant. Dauphinais has lupus, a chronic, inflammatory disease that requires her to take steroid medicines that complicate her recovery and weaken her skin and bones. "I'm a real problem child," she said. The problems, though, occur in healthy women, too.

Early on, Dauphinais switched plastic surgeons to Dr. Michael Meininger, a Wayne State University plastic surgeon, when her original doctor could not see her when she developed an infection. "It's important to have a skilled plastic surgeon because you are so vulnerable," she said. "There's no comparison to the amount of time I've spent with him, compared to my medical oncologist. Your reconstruction is much more of an art, compared to chemotherapy, which follows standardized protocols."

Meininger tried twice to make nipples for Dauphinais. The first time, in January 2013, he used fat grafted from her tummy. "They kind of looked like little worms," she recalled. Meininger tried again in May, using scar tissue to build a better nipple.

That worked a little better, but her nipples were still tiny little nubs. Dauphinais and Meininger agreed to revisit their discussion about plumping up her nipples with various new injectable medicines after she got her tattoos.

While Myers applied her inks, Dauphinais told him her reconstruction story. Myers scoffed at the mention of injectable products increasingly used in breast reconstruction to fill out the breast and the nipple. The same products are used to fill in frown lines and wrinkles. "The injectables they use for protrusion are just temporary," Myers said. "It will be

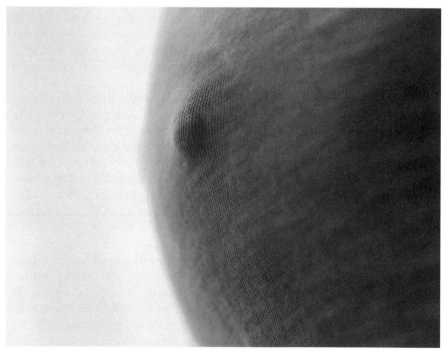

Even after nipple reconstruction surgery, many women are dissatisfied with nipples that look like tiny little nubs.

absorbed after a period of time. A doctor actually told me there's redundancy built into everything so he can continue to have you come back to do more. In this business of breast cancer they do it to make money."

Myers wasn't impressed with Dauphinais's nipples either. "This skin is too loose," he said, inspecting one closely. "The needle won't penetrate it. It won't take. I can attempt it but you'll get a mottled color around the nipple. Some of the scar tissue is hard to tattoo. The color will be slightly different. There's not much you can do about it."

They agree to leave the nipples alone and just color in the areolae. From a selection of dozens of colors, he picked some brown, red, and tan-colored bottles, into which he dipped a power tool that etches the ink into her breast. Dauphinais has no sensation in her breast, a common outcome after breast reconstruction. She didn't feel a thing. "How much will this fade?" she asked Myers. "It won't fade," he answered flatly. "It may not be quite as red later."

Five minutes later, Myers yelled "one down" to indicate he is done with one breast. He swung around the plastic black leather chair Dauphinais sat in so she could face a full-length mirror for closer inspection.

"I think that looks really good," she said. Her mother steps around to look too. "I think it looks excellent," the daughter said to her mother. "You were afraid."

Her mom replied, "Well, if you don't like it you better speak up, my dear." They laugh.

Work proceeded quickly with the second breast. Myers covered standard questions as he finished. "I've heard people say they will scab over," Dauphinais said. Myers replied, "You will get a little scabbing. It's not a heavy scab. It's kind of a light, flakey kind of scab. You apply ointment a couple times a day. You have to wear a patch at night. And if you have to wear a bra, you'll wear a patch on it."

She asked: "Am I supposed to wear a bra home?" Myers: "Yeah. I'll give you some packs of Neosporin. You may have a slight variation in the color because of the scar. There are variations in areolas too from natural ones."

Myers told Dauphinais that if she goes braless she can avoid patching her breasts for the next four or five days, but she must continue to put the cream on her breasts until any scabbing is gone.

He handed her a pink bag of supplies with patches, six packages of Neosporin cream, and a written set of instructions, including his cell phone number. "If anything goes wrong or that's out of the ordinary, bleeding, swelling, cracking or anything that doesn't look right, just give me a call. And if it's not completely healed in 10 days, give me a call."

"OK," Dauphinais told him. Her mom steps by her side again. "They look very good to me."

A few weeks later, Dauphinais saw Meininger for the discussion they postponed about making her nipples larger with injectable fillers. He agreed with Myers that the fillers "eventually will go away" but prefers that choice to enhancing her breasts with fat grafts and other methods. "The safest option is the most reasonable," he said, noting her past complications.

They also discussed that Dauphinais has developed some wrinkling in her new left breast. He raised the possibility that in the months ahead, Dauphinais could come in to have her current silicone implant exchanged for a new generation of devices. Made from a more solid type of silicone, these so-called gummy bear implants, dubbed for their consistency, offer a stronger device less prone to leakage and other problems, as occurred with past generations of implants, manufacturers say. Only some plastic surgeons offer the new implants because patients must be part of a national study to get them.

Meininger and Dauphinais agree to try injectable fillers first to address her small nipple size. She made an appointment to get the work done. A nurse practitioner in Meininger's practice gave Dauphinais a gown, told her to undress from the waist up, and returned with a small needle. Meininger checked in before the nurse started her work. "I'd stay away from this upper border where it's stiff," he said. "Go lower."

Delicately, she inserted the needle, looking for a spot without a scar. "You won't feel anything because there's a little lidocaine in it," she said, referring to the generic painkiller. She gave Dauphinais a hand mirror and said, "See how the skin is a little white here. That's where I filled the sac. I tried to widen it out" under the nipple, she said.

"I do baby steps. We can keep gradually adding until we arrive at that magic place."

She went to get Meininger to inspect her work. "We've gone through a lot of trouble for what, this?" he said, laughing.

"I think I've put in as much as I can today," she said. "I didn't want to push too hard. I was hoping for a little more." They agree Dauphinais may need a second appointment to get another dose of Juvederm, an injectable filler, a month later.

The nurse practitioner said she has been doing breast tats since 2003. "There's been a progression of the technology," she said. One year, the American Society of Plastic Surgical Nurses, a professional nursing organization of which she is a member, brought in a tattoo artist to discuss techniques. She also did a training program in areola tattooing with Rose Marie Beauchemin, founder of the Beau Institute for Permanent and Corrective Cosmetics in Mt. Laurel, New Jersey.

With time, she's also learned exactly where to inject the filler. "You look for soft edges" to place the needle so the medicine "melts into the skin." She avoids areas with scar tissue.

A month later, Dauphinais returned for another injection. The nurse practitioner asked her of the first round, "Do you think it helped?" She replied, "I think it did. I'm good for another round."

Meininger stepped in to check Dauphinais's results, and they also revisit whether she should get a new gummy-bear-type implant or fat grafting because her current implant has produced wrinkling in her left breast. "It's a roll of the dice that fat grafting will take," he said. The process, involving a liposuction-like removal of liquid fat from the abdomen and other areas, works about 60 percent of the time, he said. Newer sixth-generation implants are more durable and less prone to wrinkling and other problems, Meininger said.

That's as far as they discuss Dauphinais's options down the road. "Today, let's Juvederm your nipples," the nurse said. She stopped one injection when she noticed the skin turning white. "Let's fatten this puppy up on the other side," she said, moving to Dauphinais's right nipple.

She finishes by telling her to squeeze her nipples a little when she gets home because the filler materials are moldable for about a day.

"Nice nips," she said, closing the door as she said goodbye.

Within a few days, Dauphinais had the nipples she wanted. The filler material helped them grow and plump up.

By June 2014, Dauphinais returned for what she hoped was her last breast surgery, for a while at least.

Meininger exchanged her silicone implants for two gummy bear implants because they are considered more durable than previous ones. But within a few months, they had shifted and were painful. Meininger told her he couldn't help her further and she needed a fresh start with a new doctor.

FINANCIAL HELP FOR NIPPLE TATTOOS

The Pink Ink Fund provides $200 to $250 for any man or woman for nipple and areola tattoos after a mastectomy. It was founded by Richmond, Virginia, tattoo artist Amy Black. For details: http://pinkinkfund.org.

13

Revisionists

Donna Dauphinais was devastated. She had been trying for three years since her double mastectomy to get new breasts, and now here she was, with silicone implants that had flipped upside down inside her chest and gotten hard and painful.

When her plastic surgeon for the last three years told her there was nothing more he could do, she cried, then soon picked up the phone and made an appointment with Dr. Dennis Hammond, a Grand Rapids, Michigan, plastic surgeon with a substantial practice in fixing breast implants.

Breast revisionists are an upper tier of plastic surgeons like Hammond who devote as much as a third to half of their practice to breast reconstruction makeovers.

In medicine, these are called secondary breast revision procedures to fine-tune the first surgery but also fix implants over the years.

Often, there are three, four, five, or more procedures to revise what didn't go right the first time. One study presented in 2015 at the annual meeting of the American Society of Breast Surgeons found that 88 percent of four thousand women had at least two breast reconstruction operations, and 39 percent had four or more.[1]

Some revisionists, like Hammond, primarily are breast implants experts. They are adept in swapping out old implants for new ones using new products and techniques to improve outcomes. They often are active leaders in clinical studies of new breast implants, or implant industry consultants, giving women access to new implant designs and sizes. Other plastic surgeons bring highly advanced microsurgery skills and implant skills to reconstruct breasts. Sometimes they rebuild a breast with both implant and microsurgery techniques.

The choices bring new options for women, particularly those with D or larger bra cups, plastic surgeons say. They also are seeing middle-aged and older women in their offices who have lived for years with unsatisfying results and who finally ask themselves: Why not?

"I see women nearing retirement and they say you know what? It's time to do something for myself," said Dr. Karen Horton, a San Francisco plastic surgeon who spends nearly half of her time on breast revision surgery.

One of her patients, who was eighty-five, wanted breast reconstruction before she remarried, she said. "It's really exciting. I'm so honored to help them on the next stage of their journey. I let them know, you deserve this."

The older the woman, the guiltier she may feel about spending time and money on additional plastic surgery. "There definitely is an element of 'Oh, you should just be happy to be alive,'" Horton said. "'You have a good marriage. You aren't dating.' My feeling is, if there is something we should do, of course we should do it. Do you really want to wear that sweaty prosthesis when you are golfing, or do you want to worry about the filler coming out of your suit when you are swimming? Do you want to feel comfortable in your own skin? Many of these women have stopped looking in the mirror when they are having sex with their husband or partner. They keep the lights off. They don't even like looking at that part of their body. They feel like they've lost all their sensuality associated with being a woman that comes with their breast. I think it's definitely worth it. You are never too old."

Breast revision particularly has grown with a technique called fat grafting. It's a liposuction-like procedure in which a plastic surgeon uses a long needle to extract a woman's unwanted fat from the tummy, butt, inner thigh, or abdomen. The extracted cells are purified into a sterile liquid then injected into the breast for shape and support. Hammond, who lectures internationally on silicone implantation and revision, calls fat grafting "one of the biggest game-changers" in breast reconstruction.

"It has taken us to a whole new level," Hammond said. "This is an evolving field. We are very comfortable with large-volume fat grafting and we are very aggressive with it. Basically we do it like a standard liposuction. We use it to fill in tissue contours. That way, we can soften those contours and create a realistic-looking breast."

The reality is, breast revision is in the future of nearly every woman who gets breast implants because they aren't made to last a lifetime.

More than half of all silicone implants are replaced within ten years because they get distorted, are painful, cause exterior wrinkling, or, sometimes, fail completely, according to ten-year studies by implant manufacturers.

Four common reasons why women undergo revision surgery are, according to the plastic surgery website:[2]

- Women want smaller or bigger breasts.
- They age and they want breasts to reflect changes their bodies have made.

- Their implants have an empty appearance at the top of the bust line.
- The implant ripples, gets distorted, or hardens.

Dr. Joseph Disa, a plastic surgeon at New York City's Memorial Sloan Kettering Hospital Cancer Center, explained it this way: "Generally speaking as patients and implants age, there comes a time when a revision may be necessary because the implants fail. They may develop an implant malposition where the implant shifts. They could get capsular contracture or hard scar tissue around their implant or scar tissue that causes hardening of the implant. Or if it's a unilateral construction, their natural breast may change as they age. It may get saggy. The breast volume may change with weight changes in the patient, bigger or smaller. What looked symmetrical five or ten years ago, or twenty years ago, may not look the same today, and they come back for a revisionary operation to improve their overall aesthetics."

"I do have patients who come in to have their implants checked and they have less than ideal reconstruction. They certainly have reasons for a revision but they don't want to do it. There are other women who want to do it. Part of that is because breast cancer and breast cancer reconstruction have been in the media so much for the last several years and famous people are talking about it. That makes people think more about it perhaps."

Disa, who focuses 80 percent of his practice on breast reconstruction, with up to 30 percent of it in breast revision procedures, advises women that if their implants are not causing problems, don't tinker with them.

"If the implants are fine and the cosmetics are fine, there is no reason to change an implant. If nothing is broke, you don't have to fix it. Implant failure is uncommon. It's less than 10%, in the literature. I have to tell you that one of the less common reasons that I replace implants is not because they are broke. The most common reason I replace implants is because of the aesthetics of it, how the implant looks or feels and how it's aged over time. Patients have lost some of the symmetry they had and they are looking for a revision to make things more symmetrical and to have a little more freedom in their clothing."

For some women, getting a good-looking set of new breasts can take years.

Jill Kreifels, fifty-two, of San Jose, California, had more than a dozen procedures over eight years, reconstructing her breasts with both implants and tissue-transfer methods. She had infections after both. "It was important for me to feel like a normal person, a normal woman," she said, explaining her persistence. She said she has a medical folder that got so big it had to be broken down in separate files chronologically.

Kreifels said it took her years to accept the reality that some people's bodies, including hers, can't accept implants.

"Implants are really tricky," said Kreifels, a marketing manager for a computer company that sells electronic components. "I know a lot of people have tried to use them. I've tried to use them. But not everybody's a candidate for it. You've got to prepare yourself for that. You may get scar tissue and it makes your breasts hard." Kreifels said she liked the fact that Horton, her plastic surgeon, did not sugarcoat things for her. "She's the one who says everything up front."

In the end, Horton removed Kreifels's implants and performed a second tissue-transfer procedure in 2014. Once the breast swelling went down, she used fat grafts to shore up Kreifels's misshapen breasts. "My breasts are looking good," Kreifels said. "I'd like them to be bigger but there's not a lot I can do about that. I don't have enough fat."

Sometimes, women find that their own breast surgeons are reluctant to do more corrective procedures, if they have developed problems before.

With two previous implant failures, Donna Dauphinais was beginning to wonder if she could find a doctor to fix her problems. She sent Hammond her records and drove three hours from her Detroit-area home with her mother to see him early in 2015.

By the time of her appointment, Hammond had reviewed the medical records she sent him.

They discussed the problems she had developed, particularly pain from her distorted, hardened breast implants. Then Hammond examined her. Aware that she knows a lot about implants, down to volume sizes, he quickly talked specifics, including his recommendation that she could handle a larger implant. "I have a 750 and an 800 cc available and I'm kind of leaning toward the 750 version," he said, citing two of the largest implant sizes available.

Dauphinais answered, "It seems to make sense, if it makes sense to you. Whatever makes sense to you. You are the expert. I had the 800s. I felt they were great and all I needed was correction of the horrible ripples." Hammond responded, "The volume was OK but the ripples were the problem. So the 750s are in the ballpark then?" She said, "I'm going to leave that up to you."

To better plot the surgery and to establish baseline, presurgery measurements, Hammond and two doctors-in-training asked Dauphinais to move to a small adjacent room that Hammond called his "photo suite." It has several 3-D cameras mounted on a tripod to capture pre and post breast surgery photos, particularly breast volume. Hammond hopes the photos provide an answer to a critical question: Just how much of the fat injected into the breast remains six months later? The question frames the broader debate in plastic surgery about the value of fat grafting.

Dauphinais had no problem with the photo session. Like many women with breast cancer, she is accustomed to taking off her shirt and showing her breasts to doctors. She stood in a paper, periwinkle-blue hospital gown with a matching loincloth and posed on a small, revolving pedestal, allowing the doctors to easily move her sideways for views. She stood erect as ordered and faced the camera.

"You've got more than enough fat to graft," Hammond said. "You are going to be amazed at what we can accomplish with that fat grafting. It's real easy. So I got to tell you. I have high hopes."

Hammond took a few minutes to explain fat grafting with a video on his computer from a speech he had given at a breast cancer symposium. He was excited about the reaction he got from the talk.

The video shows a doctor inserting a large tube or cannula into a small incision in the upper thigh to obtain fat. "As we get the fat out, it will come through the tubing right here," Hammond said, pointing to the picture of fat passing through the tube.

"We'll collect it in this jar and then once we've got that fat collected we'll wash away all the debris, all the broken cells, all the fibrous tissue. There's a very simple way we do that. People just love this part. You put it through a sieve like this." He stops to show a closeup in the video of a kitchen sieve used to strain the fat. "Even better, we take a spoon and we stir it and stir it. You see what happens? All the water comes out. So we take this pH-controlled fluid—buffered saline is what it is—we pour it in here and we wash away all the debris so that what we get when this is all done is pure fat. This is a recent technological modification. There have been a bunch of little fixes to this whole process that made it a really useful procedure."

Hammond believes fat cells injected into the breast stay alive and can foster cell growth. "The astonishing thing for many surgeons is that they would expect that fat to die because it was not connected with any blood supply," Hammond said. "But because fluid is collected with it, this is a histologic specimen. Those are cells. So what it means is you can get away with a whole lot more than you think you can when it comes to fat grafting."

Hammond said he planned to use a product known generically as acellular dermal matrix, or ADM, to add support in the lower part of Dauphinais's breast.

ADM is a category of sterilized skin products, with cells removed that are used for scaffolding and shaping in the breast. Like fat grafting, ADM use is on the rise in breast revision procedures but remains under study about its effectiveness.

Research published in the January 2014 issue of *Plastic and Reconstructive Surgery* by a Georgetown University team concluded that ADM products "have proven to be a reliable tool in managing some of the most common and challenging problems in implant-based breast reconstruction."[3]

But the year before, guidelines published by two leading British breast cancer surgery and reconstruction medical groups said that concerns remain about the use of ADM products, citing higher complication rates in earlier studies. The two organizations graded them as low evidence that ADM products improve outcomes and said they support a national database to follow the issue more closely.[4]

Hammond and other doctors typically use ADM with fat grafting to add contour and support for a breast implant. He told Dauphinais that he would fill in the chest pocket that held one of Dauphinais's implants with both fat and the ADM product. But first, he would perform a cap-sulotomy, a technique to relieve the hardened scar tissue that can build around a breast implant. Hammond uses a small electrical surgery knife to remove breast tissue, causing the pocket to shrink and close a little. He also prescribes prednisone, an anti-inflammatory drug, to cut down on any inflammation caused by the new surgery. "That's another trick we have," he said.

Hammond returned to making a few final notations on Dauphinais's chest in various colored marking pens. He understands breast implants the way a hardware store owner knows his inventory.

"So we're looking at going with the smooth, round profile and a vol-ume of 750," he said, referring to one of the larger size implants available.

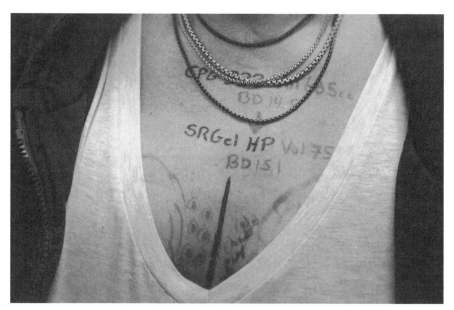

Dr. Dennis Hammond uses markings like these to plot breast reconstruction decisions.

Then, he began drawing on Dauphinais's tummy, below her belly button, as well as her inner thigh. "We're going to use a little of this fat there," he said. "That's all just my Christmas present to you. We're not going to get much fat out of there. Where we're going to get the fat from more is from your hips, like this and like this," he said, drawing circles with another marking pen. Then he returned to looking at her nipples. "My feeling here is this is not a bad attempt at a nipple. It's one of the more interesting nipples I've seen. But I think we can make it better with composite graft technology. So I think if we come down here under the arm and get this little dog ear off like this, flatten it, and we can use that to tuck in there to broaden the base out a little bit and make it look more like a natural looking nipple."

Asked to summarize Dauphinais's problems, Hammond responded, "She has asymmetry with a capsular contracture, shape distortion, and some funny-looking nipples."

Dauphinais's surgery a few days later took about four hours. Hammond emerged in scrubs from the operating room and sat in a private room in the surgery lounge to explain what happened to Dorothy Dauphinais.

"We didn't have any problems at all," he said. "I did exactly everything I said I was going to do. The implants were not ruptured. They in fact were in pretty good shape. You know what. They were flipped around. They were in completely the wrong place. The former plastic surgeon did a pretty valiant effort to get these pockets controlled. But there was just really no hope of trying to make an anatomic implant fit this pocket. So what I did was I went in and loosened everything up. I ended up putting an 800 cc implant back in. She handles that implant without any trouble at it. And then I did fat grafts. So I took fat mostly from her tummy and a little from her legs."

Dauphinais and her mother headed to a nearby hotel for the night after the surgery, then returned the next day to see staff before driving home. The recovery was tough, she said. She took a week off work while her mother helped her with basic tasks she was too sore to do, like cooking. But within a week, Dauphinais got back to a near-normal stride. It was worth it, she concluded.

"I feel better with these implants. It's like, they're happy. I feel like they are part of me. I think it's from the fat layer over it. They fit my body better. I think it's a combination of that. They just look natural. They look like they are in a natural place. My first ones were round. They were also 800 ccs. But they had a different projection so they had a smaller base. Your natural breast comes out a little farther here," she said, pointing next to the lower part of her breast.

"I feel like, it's my body."

Despite all the problems, Dauphinais said she is glad she didn't settle for less and that she had "no regrets."

Hammond still thought he could fine-tune things just a little more. Dauphinais returned six months later for a fat-grafting procedure that she hoped was her last.

14

Sex and Intimacy

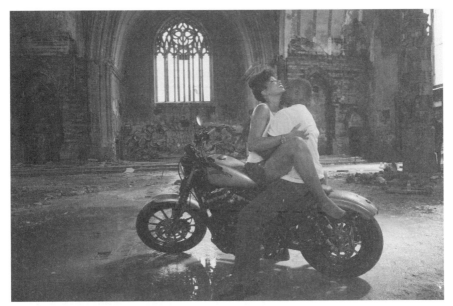

Katrina and Donald Studvent had to overcome marital and financial issues when she was diagnosed with breast cancer.

When Donald Studvent saw Katrina at a hockey bar over a Memorial Day weekend in 2003, he felt the urge to go up to the tall, striking woman and introduce himself, even though she was talking to four friends. "She really caught my attention," he said.

Katrina and Donald talked briefly and exchanged phone numbers. He called her the next day. Within a few weeks, they were talking on the phone every day, hours at a time.

"I've never been a phone man," he said. "I'm on the phone as little as possible. But with my wife, we were on the phone for hours. I want to say our record was 11 hours. We talked about everything. Life, society, religion, politics, culture, food, land, birds, astrology, history."

By July 3, Studvent couldn't wait any longer to see Katrina, who at the time was an assistant director of admissions for the Illinois Institute of Art–Chicago. She would later earn a master's in Social Work from the University of Michigan.

Donald jumped on his motorcycle and speeded to see her in Chicago, oblivious to a state trooper who "clocked me at 190" miles per hour, Studvent said. He paid a hefty fine, endured the jokes of the trooper about why he was so distracted, and got back on the road to Chicago, at a more respectable speed.

By May, they were married and soon, they had a baby.

Then, before they celebrated their second wedding anniversary, Katrina was diagnosed with stage 3 breast cancer, at age thirty, the same age of Donald's sister when she found out she had breast cancer.

The diagnosis shocked and frightened them.

What they hadn't counted on was just how tense their relationship got, as they juggled Katrina's cancer treatments with raising a young child and holding down two jobs. As common as friction like this can be, it remains a largely untouched subject for couples after a breast cancer diagnosis.

Rose Gow, fifty-seven, a high school career development counselor from Macomb, Michigan, lives with two breasts reconstructed differently that don't match. She's had several dozen procedures and still is not done. Her plastic surgeon has told her he may not be able to help her any further.

The problems made her depressed and adversely affected her marriage, she said.

"This is hard to say but my husband hasn't touched me or looked at me since," she said. "No fault to him. He doesn't know how to deal with it. He's one of those guys who do not talk about their feelings."

Reconstruction presents different challenges for single women.

Diane Mapes, a single Seattle woman and breast cancer blogger, talked frankly about being dumped by her boyfriend after her diagnosis in one post on her Double Whammied Facebook page. "While some men walk the other way, others are downright respectful," she said. "Some guys completely get what you've been through and think you are a cross between the The Big C's Laura Linney and Xena, the Cancer Warrior Princess," she wrote in a November 2011 post, referring to two TV characters. "Others would just as soon steer the conversation back to their own fascinating challenges. . . . Still others want to talk exclusively about reconstruction, as in when are you getting your new boobs and just how big are these boobs going to be. The bottom line is people are people and just because you're an official card-carrying member of the Cancer Club, it doesn't mean they're going to act any better or worse than they normally would."

Regaining intimacy, or establishing it for the first time with a new partner, may take time. Most importantly, women and experts say, women need to learn to be comfortable first with their own bodies to be a confident, supportive sexual partner.

Barbara Musser, a Petaluma, California, sex therapist and breast cancer survivor, said too many women feel like "damaged goods" after surgery. "Early on, cancer tends to define your life; it certainly did for me," said Musser, who lectures, holds workshops, and blogs frequently on the topic of sex after cancer on her website, www.sexyaftercancer.com.

"That changes after a while. Yes, my life has been shaped by my cancer experience but that's not the primary identification I have with myself. My sex appeal is not focused on what my breasts look like. My sex appeal has to do with how confident I am and how comfortable I am in my own skin. That's something that has been a gift to me from this cancer experience. When you no longer fit society's definition of what beauty is, I get to define beauty on my own terms. That's been a very important part of my journey. I work a lot with women on that: What is beautiful? What is sexy? Really, breasts may be an initial attracting factor to some men but honestly, if that's what they are focused on, they probably aren't the kind of person I want to be with."

⸺⸺》《⸺⸺

Katrina and Donald Studvent are dedicated to each other, in their eleventh year of marriage. She is thirty-nine. He is forty-seven. They are raising their daughter, ten, and his son, sixteen, while holding down two demanding careers.

Don owns and runs the 1917 American Bistro, a popular northwest side Detroit restaurant. Katrina directs the Susan G. Komen Race for the Cure–Detroit program at the Barbara Ann Karmanos Cancer Institute. She oversees Komen's annual Race for the Cure fund-raising event in the city and its affiliated community programs.

A handsome couple, they are striking in their own ways. She is tall, leggy, and stylish; he is equally tall, has an enormous hug and the voice of a broadcaster.

Katrina's diagnosis with a stage 3 breast tumor quickly upturned their lives, strained their marriage, and took months before they could return to resuming the intimacy they once had.

Katrina had a single mastectomy with a silicone implant, but she developed an infection in the expander phase of the procedure and her plastic surgeon took out the temporary implant.

She decided to live one-breasted, a decision she was comfortable with until she underwent reconstruction seven years later.

In the beginning, it frightened Donald, seeing the woman he loved so much suffer, particularly the severe side effects Katrina developed.

The couple found it easier for Katrina to live most of the week with her mother during some of the toughest first weeks. She and Donald's mother helped watched their young daughter while Katrina underwent chemotherapy.

"With my husband, everybody deals with adversity differently," Katrina said. "He was scared. So was I. Two scared people. It was a lot of conflict. A lot of friction. I had certain expectations. I'd say, because of the demands I put on him, it became difficult for us to be together at that time."

Katrina wanted support, not sympathy. "I wanted a sense of assurance from my husband that we would continue to move toward our family's future goals and not dwell on my diagnosis. You need a partner that will continue to manage the household while you are down for the count because of a chemotherapy treatment."

To juggle chemotherapy and being a mom, Katrina called on both her mom and mother-in-law for support. "I had treatments that began on Thursdays," Katrina said. "I made sure I would eat before because I knew after that I'd have no appetite. I'd be on my back until the following Wednesday. Thursday I would do chemo again. Friday, I got a shot to keep my white blood cells up. My mom picked me up and took me to her house, where I stayed until Wednesday. I was down from Sunday to Wednesday. I was sick. I couldn't deal with light. I couldn't deal with sound. Everything nauseated me. Everything going in tasted like metal. I had mouth sores. I had neuropathy. I had hot flashes. I lost my hair. And then I have this little one, thirteen-months-old, whom I can't pick up, I can't hold, I can't do for her."

Money issues also strained family dynamics. Donald was an auto assembly-line worker at the time, when the industry had mandatory plant closures and workers received only a portion of their pay.

"We were a two-income family household," Katrina said. "I was going on short-term then long-term disability, which means that our income was being cut. It was almost like going through a pregnancy when you want to get everything in order because this big thing was coming. We need to get this in order is what I was thinking. You need to get a second job because this is the income we used to have. We were in the process of looking for a house. You want your life to continue. I needed my household a certain way, going through this situation. I needed to know, who was on my team and who could handle it. And those that didn't, I didn't need that. I didn't have time to take anybody to the wayside. I had a schedule. I was blessed enough to have these people do this. I would have somebody drive me to treatment and then drop me off at my apartment. I'd drop my daughter off at my mother-in-law's house before I went to treatment."

"Then they'd drop me off, make sure I had something to eat, and I'd go lay down. I would request the TV volume to be low and limit use of lights except a little light from the kitchen. And I understood when family and friends could not adjust to my needs. It just meant you couldn't support me right now, and that's OK."

Katrina got through chemotherapy and began to resume her life. "After breast cancer you are in a new normal and it's in all areas of your life, your emotions, physical abilities, how you view yourself," she said. "Getting comfortable with that new normal is important."

Once Don Studvent saw his wife's health return, he felt relieved. "I was happier because she was alive. I was more grateful for her life than I was worried about having her breast removed."

To his wife's amusement, Studvent gave an automotive comparison to his wife's recovery. "Yes. I gave her time. When she went through everything, even with the chemo, after the chemo, it's almost as if the body is actually on a time clock, like a car with a timing belt, which keeps everything in sync and on time. Her body wasn't in sync. Her body was thrown off. It had to get itself realigned again."

Over months, they resumed their sex life. At first, Katrina felt most comfortable covering her chest, like many women. "It sounds so vain, but you question your beauty, your femininity, a lot of things," she said. "You tend to be a little shy. You want to cover. And there are some zones you don't want anyone to touch, at least not right away."

"I want to say I took a different path in the same direction," Donald said. "I had to be careful because it's so sensitive on her left side. A couple times, if I wasn't paying attention to her left side, it hurt her. You really have to be careful and really have to pay attention. I remember that. A few times, I asked to take a washcloth and just washed the left side a little bit. It can be so tender. If you apply just a little bit of pressure, it hurt her. There's still pressure after all this time."

Katrina got more comfortable with being flat-chested and joked about losing her breast form around her house. "I was always late because I couldn't find it," she laughed. "My kids would pick it up and throw it like a ball." A turning point came on a Caribbean vacation when she tried to stuff a breast form in her pink bikini. When she couldn't push the breast form "into the little triangle" top, she decided to go without the form.

"I asked my husband, how do I look? He said, 'You look fine; you look beautiful.' So I went to the pool wearing my bikini without a breast prosthesis. I was feeling a little self-conscious. A lady approached me and somehow the conversation evolved to me acknowledging I was a breast cancer survivor. I realized if someone had a question, they'd ask. And guess what? That's a way to educate them. I just started looking at it in that light, versus looking at it as a negative."

Over the years, Donald also has become equally comfortable talking to men whose partners have breast cancer. "I do talk to men about the seriousness of it for their partners and for them too," he said. "I understand there are a lot of cases where the lumps are found by the husband. I'm always talking to the fellas. I tell them, hey, play with them. Touch them because you can save a life. It's that serious."

In 2013, Katrina decided to return for reconstruction. "When I went back for reconstruction, it wasn't a matter of, 'oh my God, I must do this.' It was more, 'why not?' I approached it in a way like some people do this because they want bigger breasts. I'm here, minus one. Why not? If it takes, great. If not, I'll leave it alone. It took."

Her plastic surgeon, Dr. Michael Meininger, of Birmingham, Michigan, inserted one silicone implant in her left breast and a smaller one on her healthy right side. He attempted nipple reconstruction but it failed, so she has a nipple and areola on her right breast and a tattooed areola and no nipple on the left.

Otherwise, her breasts "match somewhat," she said. "They do the job; they fill out the shirt. I'm pleased with them."

Still, she added, "It's never the same. I don't care what everyone says. I notice that with weight gain they change. The right one got a little larger than the left. You can see a significant difference. I had a lift but there's still some sagging there, still some drooping. The left side, it's all implant. It's firmer."

"I do not have all the feeling back under my arm. There's some tissue scarring there. I have more feeling than I expected. Most people are fully numb there. It doesn't hurt. There was a period I was just numb and didn't feel anything. You learn to live with it and the reason why is I went years without one. I went from nothing to at least I now have something, some cleavage. It looks a little more normal than the prosthesis did. In that respect it's a lot different."

Donald Studvent thinks cancer liberated his wife and changed the balance of their relationship, for the better.

"I always tell people I am a true cave man. I like cars, trucks and anything greasy and challenging. For me, I was really more concerned about her happiness and about her being satisfied. My wife is a little bit conservative. I think the older I get the more conservative I am. I think we are switching roles. When I met her, she was more conservative. Now she's more on the edgy side and I'm more conservative."

He likes to tell other men that "life is more important than the breast. You can grow old with your loved one. Remember that life is more important than the breast. That's the best advice I can give, to make sure that you have a long, healthy life. If it's agreed upon and there's reconstruction, make sure that person doesn't have any stress and you are supportive. You can always get another breast. You can't get another life."

In 2015, the Studvents resumed a discussion they postponed about having another child. It would require in-vitro fertilization, which is time consuming and has a higher chance of resulting in multiple embryos and possibly pregnancies.

"I'm on the fence," Katrina said. "The shots, taking time out of your schedule. I don't know if I can commit to that yet, even though I want a baby. And then, what if there's two babies instead of one? I'm terrified. They would be two against one. They'd tackle me. But we have to make a decision. I'll be 40 next year. The fertility doctor says there are some sobering statistics" about how much harder it gets, she said.

Pregnancy, sex, and intimacy are important issues to younger women with breast cancer, she said. "Some of these women are under 40, starting to have children or they have young children. It's a challenge. Your body has changed tremendously."

"I think everything starts with you loving you. If you love you, then you become more comfortable with others and that confidence you need comes through. Most men want a confident lover. Most men don't want someone who is unsure. But if you are unsure, I would hope that whomever you have this relationship with is engaging enough to be a support. But it starts with you becoming OK with you, and that new normal."

Katrina wishes more women heard about the positives that can follow a breast cancer diagnosis. "People tell you the grit. You'll have a scar. Here are the basic things that are going to happen. But no one ever says what happens after breast cancer. You aren't dying. You are living. You are going through this treatment to live. So your quality of life has changed but it hasn't changed to the point where you can't go on. Life is good. I wish someone had given me a glimpse at that silver lining, other than saying you'll make it out of surgery."

REVIVING INTIMACY

Sex therapist and breast cancer survivor Barbara Musser offers tips for couples interesting in rebuilding intimacy after a cancer diagnosis. She hosts a periodic blog, "Sexy Saturdays," as well as workshops. Her website, www.sexyaftercancer.com, lists events, past blog entries, videos, and a way to reach her with questions. She also offers Skype telephone sessions for people outside the San Francisco area. In an interview, she summarized some of her suggestions.

MIRROR EXERCISE

I suggest women start to look at their faces with a hand-held or bathroom mirror. They need to do this practice for 30 days for five minutes a day. The reason for the 30 days is you want to create a new neural pathway in your brain and that's what it takes to get that started. Set a timer for five minutes and look into your eyes and say the words out loud, "I love you." It's really hard for women to do that because most of us don't look at ourselves except when we are getting ready for something in the morning. So for many women, this is the first time they really deeply connect with themselves. This practice brings up everything that gets in their way. All the judgments, all the stories, all the pain, all the separation; it comes right up. It's challenging to do that. If they stick with it, they will begin to experience a shift before that 30 days are up.

The next phase is to stand and look at yourself in a full-length mirror with your clothes on, in a pretty outfit you like. Tell yourself, "I love you and you're beautiful." You do that for 30 days.

The next phase, you stand naked in front of a full-length mirror and you say, "I love you and you are beautiful." Some women can do the naked in front of the mirror exercise immediately. Many cannot. It's too confronting, too overwhelming. So I suggest easing into it. If they've done those two phases of practices, they have helped to reestablish a loving relationship with themselves. Any time you do this is ideal.

The thing about the mirror work is that often it can be a doorway into the grief and the sadness of the pain and the loss. Every woman I've talked to, there's grief inside, about the loss of a breast or part of one; grief about the loss of beauty; and the fear that comes with cancer. So there are a lot of feelings in there and many women would rather just bury them deep inside of themselves.

REDEFINE SEX

Sex is more than intercourse. If you take the letters SEX and turn it into an acronym, it may be SEX stands for Sensual Energy Exchange or Sacred Energy Exchange. What does that mean? It opens the horizon beyond genital intercourse because there are a lot of ways to exchange sexual energy. For example, sit with your partner and put on some soft background music. Hold hands, look into each other's eyes, and don't talk and breathe. There's an exchange that happens there that is very deep, very intimate. Often, people have intercourse because they want that kind of connection. Now, I'm not saying intercourse is not fun. It is. But honestly if you look at the length of time of the average sexual experience, the foreplay, the getting naked, the insertion, the orgasm, the actual inserting and orgasm part is like maybe two to three minutes, but that's where we put all the focus. My aim is to get people to expand their focus. There are other ways of finding pleasure. Then when they are ready to have intercourse again or some kind of insertion, then they are not so focused on it and people don't have to freak out about it.

GETTING IT GOING AGAIN

If you stop having sex, and it has gone on for a very long time, then you have a gap and you need to bridge that gap. One way is to build up the intimacy. Take a walk and hold hands. I also recommend that when you both get home at the end of your day, have a 30-second kiss. Not just a little peck on the cheek. With 30 seconds, you can put arms around each other, you are kissing, breathing together and getting yourself in sync with each other after the day you've both had. It starts to open your hearts to each other.

MAKE A PLEASURE MAP

Take some time, a half hour or hour, be alone, go in the bedroom, take your clothes off and you map say, the woman's body first. She lies on her tummy, naked on the bed, and he starts at her feet and he moves up her leg. He's using different types of touch. He might use his fingernails lightly going up her leg. He may do gentle massage and she gives him feedback. She might say, "When you get up half-way up my calf, I like the fingernails there, inside my leg. That feels really good." He's making some notes mentally or on a poster board. Then he goes farther up her thighs, around her buttocks, and up her back and neck. You are learning the new territory. Our bodies change as our sensations change. We may not have known these places before. Then in another session, you can have her on her back and do the same thing on her front. Then in another session you can focus on her vulva and genitals internally and externally. Then you do the same with him. It's a way of communicating with each other, and getting to know what's good, where it's numb or painful. So you know the places that feel good and then you can focus on that. A lot of people don't know how to communicate about sex. They don't know the language or they are embarrassed. This is a way to ease into that.

HAVE A WEEKLY SEX DATE

Let's pull out our pleasure map. Let's focus on kissing the neck. Take it slow. Take it easy. See what feels good. Play around. Talk about it. I also recommend taking off clothes, getting in bed, facing each other, and you have no agenda other than being together. You breathe, look into each other's eyes and see what inspires the two of you. It may be simply breathing and looking into each other's eyes. It may be pillow talk, or stroking each other's body. Maybe it's a massage. Maybe it's trying intercourse. Whatever feels right to both of you, you go with that. As long as it feels good you kept doing it. It's allowing yourself to see what's actually happening instead of this whole conversation that she may be having in her head, like he wants to have intercourse and I'm not ready for that. She may be scared. He may think, I don't want to touch her because I'm afraid I'm going to hurt her. Pretty soon, they are having separate conversations in their head instead of actually with each other. The whole idea is to be present with each other and find the places where you do connect.

15

Lymphedema

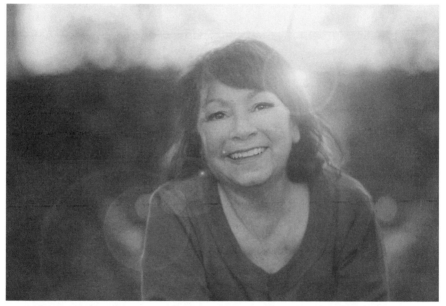

Sharon Sheffield had such severe arm and chest pain from lymphedema that she had to get therapy from a specialist.

One thing for sure, Sharon Sheffield got a great new set of breasts after her 2010 double mastectomy with saline implant reconstruction.

She likes them. Her plastic surgeon loves them.

"I told him, they may look great but they are killing me," said Sheffield, sixty, a nurse who lives in St. Charles, Illinois.

After a lumpectomy failed to give her clear margins around her tumor, Sheffield chose mastectomy. She found the expander phase of implant reconstruction "total misery" but hoped the pain would be relieved immediately when her expanders were swapped out for permanent ones.

"I remember going in to get the expanders out and I was the happiest patient I thought they ever had seen because I thought that would be the end of my pain," she said. "I remember waking up and there was no change. I was in enormous pain."

Sheffield developed postmastectomy pain syndrome, a cluster of neurological problems that caused her such severe pain "it almost took my breath away," she said.

Postmastectomy pain is pain lasting more than three months after surgery, in the chest wall, armpit, or upper arm. "It was so bad it made me almost suicidal," Sheffield said. "I thought, I can't live like this."

A nerve pain medicine, gabapentin, "seemed to help some." Some doctors also report improvements with drug cocktails of nerve block and steroid medicines.

The problems were so great that Sheffield and her husband, John, "were both depressed," she said. "I was very depressed once I realized it was not going away."

Her husband tried to get her spirits up and took her to all her medical appointments. The pain grew less intense, gradually, and Sheffield got

WHAT IS LYMPHEDEMA?

The lymphatic system is a network of tiny, thin tubes that carry a nutrient-rich lymph fluid. These vessels travel through a web of nodes, or small, round masses that store white blood cells and filter bacteria. Lymph fluid helps the body fight infection and removes fluid that leaks out of blood vessels. To stay healthy, the lymph system must keep moving. When lymph nodes are damaged or removed, scar tissue can form and keep fluid from draining.

WHO IS AT RISK?

Any woman undergoing an axillary dissection, sentinel node biopsy, or radiation is at risk. It occurs in 7 percent of women undergoing sentinel lymph node biopsy and up to about 45 percent of women undergoing axillary node dissection. Postsurgical radiation therapy increases the likelihood of arm lymphedema further. A woman's risk of lymphedema depends on her surgery, where the tumor was removed, the number of lymph nodes removed, and personal healing factors.

HOW IS IT DIAGNOSED?

Usually, a diagnosis is based on a physical exam. A test called lymphoscintigraphy can be performed to diagnose lymphedema, though it is not usually considered necessary. It involves an injection of a radioactive dye between the web spaces of the fingers that traces the lymphatic system.

LYMPHEDEMA SYMPTOMS

- Swelling in the arms, hands, fingers, shoulders, or chest.
- A feeling of heaviness or tightness in the arm.
- Restricted range of motion.
- Aching or pain.
- Decreased flexibility in the hand or wrist.
- Hardening and thickening of the skin on the arm.

Once lymphedema develops, the affected arm is susceptible to more swelling. Patients should take precautions by avoiding cuts, scratches, burns, blood pressure cuffs, and blood draws on the affected body part, as practical.

THERAPY

Certified lymphedema specialists offer specialized physical and occupational therapy. Therapists perform lymphatic massage and help women learn exercises, including arm elevations. They also can do special types of multilayer banding and help relieve lymphedema. Mechanical pumps that drain fluids also may be used.

PREVENTION

- Regularly use moisturizers to keep the skin from breaking down.
- Wear gloves during gardening.
- Avoid blood draws and blood pressure cuffs on the affected side.
- Wear compression garments during air travel.
- Wear loose jewelry and clothing.

back to her life. She returned to work as a part-time admissions nurse at a suburban Chicago hospital and started to feel more like herself again.

Then in December 2014, she decided to take an extended trip abroad with her husband. She developed lymphedema, a problem separate from the postmastectomy pain syndrome.

Lymphedema associated with breast cancer can follow surgery, lymph node dissection, radiation, or cancer itself. It causes pain and swelling in the arm, breast, chest wall, or neck. It occurs when the body's lymphatic system, a companion network to the circulatory and immune systems that trap bacteria and other germs, is injured and fluids back up within the lymphatic fluid. Overuse and underprotection of a limb from sun, infection, and other problems can cause lymphedema, as can extended air travel from low-air-compression cabins on airplanes.

Sheffield never had lymphedema before. But on one leg of her travels, she forgot the compression sleeve she normally wore. Back home, her arm severely swollen, she looked for a specialist to help.

Susan Santilli, the certified lymphedema specialist Sheffield sought out, works in the outpatient rehabilitation department at Edward-Elmhurst Healthcare, a hospital in Naperville, Illinois. An occupational therapist for thirty-eight years, Santilli has seen many forms of lymphedema. Sheffield told her that her lymphedema pain was so bad it "feels like you have a super, super tight band around your chest that you want to take off but can't." Sheffield also had developed a problem known as cording, when scar tissue forms around lymph vessels and can cause discomfort and arm tightness.

"She said she could feel it cracking underneath when she was working it," Sheffield said. "It's probably the most pain relief I've ever had. Once she started with me, I started feeling a lot of relief. My left armpit and side felt like they had metal plates in them. She broke up all that scar tissue until it felt like normal. She does massage. But she does lymphedema massage, which is real gentle, because the vessels are so close to the surface. She's probably been the most help to me."

Santilli said cording is fairly common in her patients. She explained it this way: "If you or I want to reach to the side or above our head, we do, with ease. The breast surgery patient who has cording feels like the rubber band or rope won't stretch far enough so they can't reach what they want to reach. It can be totally eradicated by doing therapy. Sometimes it comes about because the patient uses the arm too much or too soon."

Cording "can radiate all the way down to the thumb and index finger areas if it's pretty extensive," Santilli said. "It can come back. I've had patients come back and say, now look where it is. The good news is it reverses fairly quickly. I use a manual technique, working on the tissue itself, in combination with teaching the patient certain stretching exercises. And most importantly I talk to them about what not to do."

At its worst, Sheffield rated her pain a 10 on a standard 1 to 10 scale, with 10 being the worst. "I could hardly function," she said. "Later, it went to a seven when I started therapy. Now it's a two or a three."

Sheffield still doesn't like to wear bras because they hurt too much to wear, she said. "No bra for me," she said. "I wear clothing that's not very sheer." Car seat belts hurt still, she said. "Any pressure" on her chest hurts, she said.

By June 2015, Sheffield emailed to say that she rated her pain at "about a one and on some days zero! My arm is still a little swollen. I have a compression sleeve to wear when I am going to be really active, like gardening, but I must admit to not being too good with it." She also still takes gabepentin once a day for pain.

Looking back, she said, "I wish I would have known that this pain syndrome could happen. It needs to be out there," she said. "I don't think it's discussed. It alters your life terribly. That's a biggie."

Surgerywise, she's done. "I will never have reconstruction again. I would just have my breast removed and go with a prosthesis. Another surgery would cause more scar tissue. I am stuck with them. They are here and they are going to stay. I don't want any more surgeries. I didn't have nipples put on. I didn't want anyone to touch me with a knife."

———⊲⟨◍⟩⊳———

Fortunately, there is more help available, particularly for lymphedema.

Many large academic health systems have rehabilitation and therapy programs to prevent, diagnose, and treat lymphedema and postmastectomy pain, said Dr. Eric Wisotzky, who is a cancer rehabilitation and lymphedema expert and director of oncology rehabilitation for the MedStar National Rehabilitation Network, a regional network in the greater Washington, D.C., area. He is the coeditor of *Managing Breast Cancer: A Guide to Living Well Through Physical Medicine and Rehabilitation* and coauthor of the lymphedema chapter.[1]

"At many academic institutions, this is becoming a fairly well-integrated part of the program," he said. "There is a range of quality in the programs, but many institutions are offering this, and certainly some of the more comprehensive, private-practice type programs will have services available. I still have people come to us from some remote areas of the country where many of these issues are not addressed and unfortunately come to us when the situation has gotten quite severe when it might have been dealt with preemptively at an earlier stage."

Not every breast cancer patient who has surgery is at high risk of lymphedema, Wisotzky said. "That's a misunderstanding that comes up all the time." Risks are higher for women who have undergone significant lymph node dissection and radiation, he said.

Women who have had a lymph node dissection compared to those who have a less invasive sentinel lymph node biopsy have a 20 to 30 percent lifetime risk of having lymphedema, Wisotzky said.

"Radiation adds about another 10% to their risk. The most common time for lymphedema to start is six to twelve months after surgery, but many women still develop lymphedema as much as three to five years after surgery," he said. "Lymphedema becomes less common after five years, but still can occur," he said.

Overweight patients have the highest risk of the problem. "There's a great deal of evidence in the literature about that," he said. "The body's lymphatic system doesn't like fat. Certainly I tell my patients, get yourself in the best shape of your life to help prevent lymphedema."

Preoperative appointments can pinpoint lymphedema risks and help educate women about how to spot problems and what to do when one occurs, he said.

"We find out if they have any pre-existing problems with their function that potentially could impair their recovery from breast cancer, whether they had some previous neck or shoulder problem that might start acting up after surgery," he said. "Or do they have a nerve problem related to diabetes or something else that could get worse with chemotherapy treatment? We can check their arms to see if they are at risk for lymphedema and if it does occur, hopefully we can pick it up at a very early stage before it gets really bad. I think having this pre-operative assessment, having what we call pre-habilitation, at an early stage can prevent them from having a lot of the post-operative complications, or if they do get them, they are at an early stage."

Postsurgery, Wisotzky recommends arm exercises, which were once discouraged, he said, as well as skin care and sunburn protection.

Moderate-intensity exercises "have been shown to be beneficial," he said. "We also counsel people on skin care and hygiene and trauma to the skin that can precipitate lymphedema. We talk about nail care and skin care and avoiding sunburn. Use common sense precautions when doing activities that can cut the skin such as gardening. Beyond that, there are a lot of common recommendations out there in the lymphedema literature, but the truth of the matter, there's not a lot of areas with good evidence. There are a lot of gray areas. For me, I've gone away from telling patients a lot of stuff they shouldn't do. There's not a lot of good scientific evidence and I really want my patients to live their lives unrestricted. They are constantly reminded of their cancer and their fear of it. I would like to get rid of that fear and help them get back to feeling they are living a normal life. I certainly don't want to give them a recommendation that would discourage them from exercising, being active, going back to work or not trying to feel whole again."

Compression garments come in so many styles and types "that it can be confusing," so he recommends women see certified fitters for their products. The products also can run several hundred dollars each and "insurance is often a barrier," he said. "Typically Medicare and Medicaid don't cover garments. Private insurance, sometimes do cover and sometimes don't." He added, "I work in an inner-city community where many of my patients find a standard compression garment unaffordable. Garments typically need to be changed out every six months. It can be a considerable expense."

Some pain issues, particularly regarding shoulder motion, "are well addressed by the surgical team," he said. "But some of the more specific pain syndromes often are not well addressed. Oftentimes these pain syndromes are treated with medications. We don't want to deny someone pain relief. But frankly, from my perspective as a rehabilitation specialist, to me the vast majority of the time, these pain syndromes are treatable through the right rehabilitation technique. It takes a specialist in the musculoskeletal and neuro-muscular systems to evaluate these patients and to determine what the specific source of their pain is and come up with a rehabilitation plan that will address that, and hopefully it might cure that patient and they won't need to be on pain medications for the rest of their lives. Unfortunately, I see people years out and nobody's ever examined their shoulder to figure out what's going on and they've been taking pills all these years."

Some top centers offer a procedure called Vascularized Lymph Node Transfer. It replaces damaged lymph nodes with healthy ones taken elsewhere in the body, often the groin or even the neck. Doctors in San Antonio and New Orleans report permanent or substantial relief for many surgery patients. Wisotzky cautioned that the surgery is in its early days and should only be an option for women who first sought conventional therapy.

16

Arab Culture

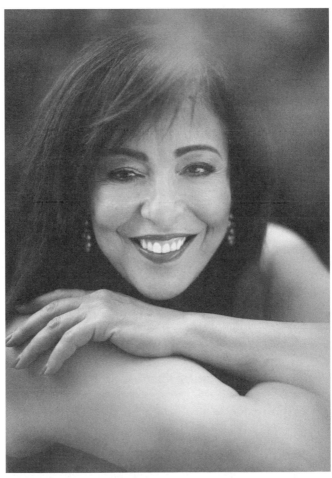

Hiam Hamade is a breast cancer survivor who shares her story with other Arab women so they know what to expect with breast reconstruction.

Here in one of the largest Arab communities in North America, a cancer diagnosis and subsequent decisions about surgery and reconstruction can bring shame, marital discord, and depression.

Just ask Hiam Hamade, who has made it her career to coax other Arab women into having mammograms, biopsies, and breast cancer surgery and reconstruction, if that's their choice.

All too often, there are obstacles to care, particularly among those who can't read, write, or speak much English. They may be immigrants and refugees from countries where cancer is diagnosed late, leaving families thinking little can be done.

For them, cancer can bring shame and stigma that can affect the entire family, and there's often a high level of secrecy, research has found.[1]

"In the Arab community, many people don't want to be recognized as cancer survivors," said Hamade, sixty-two, a mother of four and a breast cancer survivor. "They don't want to announce it. People are afraid it will be in their families, in their daughters. Or they don't want to show they have problems with their breasts. So they try their best not to show their feelings. They don't even show their husbands. They say, 'no, my husband didn't see it.' They are so scared."

Hamade coordinates a breast and cervical cancer-screening program at ACCESS, headquartered in Dearborn, Michigan, one of the largest human services organizations serving Arabs in North America.

A decade of hard work has made inroads. More women are getting mammograms. Model language translation programs are in place. Other important changes have been made, including a new generation of Arab physicians such as Dr. Majd Aburabia, the first Arabic breast surgeon for the Dearborn-based Oakwood Healthcare system. She sees families much more willing to discuss breast cancer surgery options and genetic testing.

At the same time, the nation's Affordable Care Act covers mammography, eliminating a major insurance problem in the past.

The lessons from the Arab community bring model approaches to developing culturally sensitive, hospital-based outreach programs. They demonstrate the importance of comprehensive, community-based breast cancer screening programs to breast reconstruction awareness efforts.

Here, too, are some of the first published interviews with Arab women undergoing breast cancer surgery and reconstruction. Their insights explain how culture affects a woman's body image and surgery choices.

———————————————

Hiam Hamade considers her cancer story "quite simple." She got a mammogram. It found cancer. She told her doctor she wanted a lumpectomy because she thought it would help her stay much like she was. Many Arab women like her don't want a mastectomy, she and others say.

No mastectomy for her. But she was called back twice by her doctor for additional surgery because she did not have margins free of cancer where they removed her tumor.

"The third time, I said to myself, maybe I don't trust them," Hamade recalled. She scheduled a second opinion with another doctor, who also told her to have another lumpectomy. This time, she said no.

Hamade decided to have a unilateral mastectomy with a TRAM flap, with her breasts reconstructed with her abdominal tissue. Peace of mind came first, she said. So did picking the most natural method to reconstruct her breasts. "I don't like to put something that is not mine in my body," said Hamade, a Jehovah's Witness. "Even things like Botox. I said my tissue is the best. I can't trust anything else. I love my body. I want to look decent."

"They did a very good job. They even made nipples for me. I am very satisfied. I am very happy with the results. At least I have my breasts. I love my body. I want to look as good as I can. If I have a chance to do it, why not?"

At ACCESS, Hamade freely shares her story with other women, as part of taking away their fear and misconceptions.

"One of my clients was scared," she recalled. "She was stage 2. She wanted to keep her breast. The doctor told her to have a lumpectomy. I told her my story. She was so scared to do surgery. I said to her, look, people pay big money for liposuction and things like that. You'll be OK. She was very satisfied. Now it's been seven years. When she comes to the clinic she hugs me and thanks me and says, 'You saved my life.'"

ACCESS has translated into Arabic a range of information materials, including "Arab Woman's Guide to Breast Cancer" and "Hereditary Breast Cancer: Family History is the Key," besides a shower card explaining steps to do breast self-exams.

Hamade or her assistant, Ghada Aziz, call every woman diagnosed with breast cancer through the ACCESS program and follow them through critical stages of surgery decisions. The program serves a large number of refugees and immigrants from the Middle East who need extra help with translation and navigation help through large health systems.

"We tell her what she should expect and what the surgeries are and what questions she may want to ask," Hamade said. "We do this as a volunteer job on the side. We take calls in the evenings and on the weekends. We get them to their appointments. We stand with them and we educate them as much as we can."

She sees far too many women rush to judgment, the reason she advocates pre-surgery talks with advocates like her. "She needs to be counseled before she goes to surgery. If they go straight to the doctor, the surgeon may not give them choices. The patient feels if she waits more, she will be dying of cancer. So she doesn't give herself a chance to look for resources. She rushes and she does what the surgeon says. And if they have to go back" for a revision, "they think, why should I go through this trouble again?"

Doctors and hospitals also need to spend more time helping women understand how surgery may help them. "Every doctor should give patients choices," she said. "They shouldn't say I'm scheduling you for surgery now. The women say, I'm dying, why should I have surgery? They don't know the questions to ask. The doctors sometimes don't take time to discuss options with the patient. They should. Women come a year later" after a mastectomy "and I say, why didn't you do reconstruction? They say, nobody told me."

————— ((◉)) —————

Ghada Aziz, fifty-two, was diagnosed in 2009 with an early-stage breast cancer.

She has an extensive family history of cancer. When she was fourteen, her mom died at forty years of age, three years after her breast cancer diagnosis. A sister and an aunt are breast cancer survivors.

That history made her an advocate of mammography. "I started to do mammograms when I was 30," said Aziz. "At that time, back in the eighties, I had no health insurance. So I went to the free clinics. I lived in West Virginia for 11 years. I came to Detroit and had health insurance through my work, thank God. I continued to get mammograms."

"In December 2009, I had a mammogram and they found something suspicious so for two years I had to go get another mammogram every six months. They couldn't find anything on my mammogram."

A biopsy also found nothing, but Aziz persisted and asked for a magnetic resonance imaging test, or MRI. The test found early stages of breast cancer. "We talked to the doctor and he said, 'You don't need a mastectomy. It's very small. We'll do lumpectomy and radiation.'" She had the surgery and underwent a form of internal radiation called brachytherapy. She returned to work soon and went on with her life.

Three years later, "I was doing my breast self-exam and I found a lump again in the same breast, my left, beside the nipple. I could feel it very good. My daughter felt it. I went to the doctor, who said I need to do a biopsy. They said it might be from the radiation. They did an ultrasound-guided biopsy. She said, it doesn't seem serious. It's mostly from the radiation. At that time, I thought, very good. What was scaring me was I didn't want to get it in my other breast. I remembered what my mother went through."

"I met with the surgeon and I explained to him my medical history. He said OK. He said, 'This is a decision for you.' I said, 'I want a double mastectomy.' That's what I requested from the beginning. I don't want to get the disease again. He said there still would be a chance I could get cancer in the chest wall. He gave me a choice. I said I don't want the silicone because I have a phobia for the silicone. I need something from my natural body and he said, OK, we'll do that."

Aziz developed low blood pressure and needed to wait six more months to be strong enough for surgery. She underwent a TRAM flap in August 2012, only to develop complications.

The flap of abdominal tissue placed in her left breast failed and had to be removed. She carried around a machine for weeks afterward to drain the blood and fluids oozing from her surgical drains and abdominal incision site.

"They said, you will have to wait a year and we'll do it again but we can't take it from the stomach. We'll do it from the shoulder muscle. They explained it all to me." She agreed to wait. "I want to get my health back. I don't want to go through another surgery."

By August 2013, she underwent another flap procedure. She looks better, but she has no nipples and her breasts don't perfectly match, she said.

"I want to be honest with you. It doesn't bother me. But when I get my health back, now I'm thinking maybe I'll do it, the rest of the reconstruction. I buy many bras. Inside me I wish this one was the same size as the other one so I'd look nice. It's occurred to me many times to go back to the doctor for this one (pointing to her right breast). This side is hurting me." She wears a girdle or similar compression garment all day at work to hold in her breasts and immediately takes it off when she gets home from work. It's a relief to get the garment off, she said.

Fear of more complications has kept her from going back so far.

"I'm not done. I'm still thinking about it. I think I have to do it because I'm aging and it would be harder to do when I'm older. I'd like to. But I have fear. I've been through a lot."

Aziz also sees preferences for lumpectomy among Arab women. They approach the issue of mastectomy versus lumpectomy differently, she said. "They are so scared. They don't want to talk about it. They are confused. They don't know what to do. And because of their husbands, they accept lumpectomy. I give my example to them so they have an idea about how they can take tissue. Some women accept mastectomy. Some refuse. It depends on how they are educated."

"I have a woman now who had a lump in her breast that was very suspicious to the doctor. This woman gave me a very hard time because the doctor told her that it seems to be nothing but it's better to do a biopsy. She refused to do a breast biopsy. She didn't want a needle going through her body. I explained to her. Listen, I did that five or six times in my life. You will not feel it. But she doesn't want to tell her son, her mom, or her sister. It scares them. She doesn't want her son or sister to worry about her."

"So I told her, I'll take you to the biopsy and bring you back. I said, don't worry. You won't feel anything because of the anesthesia. She was fine, doing good. I took her home. She spent Saturday and Sunday at home. I called her and she was fine. It was benign. But every year, she now gets a mammogram."

———————⮞«⦿»⮜———————

Oakwood Healthcare serves metro Detroit's Arab community with an extensive system of language and cultural outreach services.

The hospital can arrange translation services in 150 languages, particularly through one Hispanic and three Arabic translators who "do much more than interpretation," said Mohamad Rustom, director of multicultural health and clinical language services at Oakwood. "Our interpreters act as our cultural brokers. They facilitate communication between the providers, the person and the family."

For its large Muslim population, Oakwood has Halal meals; a TV channel for prayer recitations; a visiting Imam; and even a card that orients patients where to stand in the hospital, facing Mecca.

Accommodating large families of hospital visitors, as is custom in the community, can be challenging but important, Rustom said. "This is where cultural responsiveness comes in," he said. "They have a big family and need a bigger family room. We also taught the staff to pick out a spokesperson for the family, the person with the most impact. Perhaps the elderly son or lady. We have them talk to the rest of the family. People respond very positively to that. Once you have the respect piece, if you are addressing any problems, I'll follow the rules you set down for us."

Oakwood has created many culturally sensitive pieces of literature for Arab patients and their caregivers. One of them, "Provider's Guide to the Arab-American Patient," has many helpful suggestions and insights, particularly about the importance of family, hope, and optimism in the community. Some of its suggestions include:

- Arab American patients need to develop personal relationships with a health care provider before sharing personal information.
- Arab American patients are sensitive to the courtesy and respect they are accorded, and good manners are important in evaluating a person's character. Therefore, greetings and inquiries about well-being are important.
- Arab American patients value privacy and resist disclosure of personal information to strangers, especially when it relates to familial disease conditions.

- Individuals are protected from bad news as much as possible.
- Convey hope and optimism. The concept of false hope is not meaningful to Arabs because they regard God's power to heal as infinite.
- Communicating a grave diagnosis is often viewed as cruel and tactless because it deprives the patient of hope. Similarly, preoperative instructions are believed to cause needless anxiety and complications. For Muslim patients, the guide points out these rituals and food limitations:
  - Muslim patients may refuse to eat non-Halal meat or ask about food preparation.
  - Ramadan, the Muslim month of fasting, requires abstinence from eating, drinking, and smoking during daylight hours. Medicine schedules must accommodate fasting requirements.

Aburabia, a breast surgeon who joined the Oakwood system in 2009 as its first female Arabic breast surgeon, said she takes time from the beginning of a woman's first appointment to create a lasting relationship. Many seek her out as a woman. She tries to accommodate their requests if they ask that their entire health care team be female too.

"Now many women say, 'I want the best. I don't care if it's a man or a woman,'" she said. "So they are like every other woman in that regard. I've had some say I'd rather have a female, even women of white European ancestry. I have learned not to assume. I ask."

She advises staffers to knock on patient doors and to not expose a woman with cancer to others in the room if the patient must disrobe. She holds up a sheet to shield them from seeing a woman being examined.

"When I am examining a teenager, even if her mother is in the room, I have to lift the gown so they are not seeing anything," Arurabia said. "And when the family is there, you distribute your eye contact around the room, to the family present too. You do that with every woman. You figure out where she is, both medically and psycho-socially."

Aburabia raises the issue of genetic testing with women with an extended family history of cancer. Women from the near and Middle East, Latin America, and the Caribbean have higher rates of genetic mutations when testing includes broader genetic panels, she said, citing results from Myriad Genetics.[2]

Increasingly, Aburabia said she is finding Arab women willing to be tested. "Every Arab American woman I mention testing to is fully on board with it," she said. "They say, if there's any way it will help my daughter, I will do it."

By comparison, Aburabia and Rustom both have encountered Arab and other ethnic families who don't want to inform an elderly member she has breast cancer. "Everybody in the family knows except grandma," she said. "Ethically, we can't do that. You don't want to antagonize the family. But you can't do what they ask and so you say, I'm going to explain things gently to grandma. The families understand. They find out grandma knew all along."

"There's a huge need, not just women of ethnic backgrounds, but for all women to have psychological support for breast cancer. Breast cancer is different than other cancers. For most women, it's an easily curable disease. It's highly curable but it's a very cruel disease. It's cruel because it tries to take away from you the essence of what you consider being a woman means. It tries to take away your hair. It takes away your breasts or tries to. If they are on chemo, their nails can turn black or their skin suffers. It's like they aged 10 years in those couple months on chemo. So it's cruel. It changes how you look or tries to at least. But it's curable. Seeing and navigating a woman through this is hugely significant and important and time consuming. The challenge for us as clinicians is we don't have that time. You crunch constantly for time. And you need trained psychologists and psychiatrists to handle this and they are not that easy to find. And is there insurance coverage for that? Those are huge barriers."

Families also need to be included in health care decisions, said Dr. Haythem Ali, a medical oncologist in the Henry Ford Health System, Detroit. Often, Arab families "circle their wagons to protect the ill person from anything they perceive to be harmful to them, including the knowledge of them having cancer."

"It's almost as if they feel the information is as harmful as the disease itself. Sometimes I have talked about these issues without using certain words. But it's very, very difficult. When you are talking about chemotherapy, which is a harsh therapy with side effects, I find you need to have a lot of knowledge about the illness in order to become an ally of the physician, not an adversary. You can't make an ally from someone who doesn't know what you are doing. If she thinks you are doing things to her, rather than her doing things with you, then it's almost impossible to get a good conversation."

⟫⟪◉⟫⟪

Adnan Hammad is a PhD health educator and executive director of the North American Arab Medical Association, a nonprofit organization that provides educational and medical resources to Arabs throughout the world. He developed the ACCESS health program, and early on, he even went door to door to survey one Arab neighborhood about attitudes toward mammography. He found more than half of the women never got the tests. Hammad then applied for a $30,000 state grant to provide mammography services to Arab women.

One problem: in the beginning, no one wanted to get one. "The first three months, we scheduled women for mammograms and no one was going," Hammad said.

Some thought it was surgery. Even the few Hiam Hamade coaxed in to get the test got scared about subsequent biopsy tests needed to confirm a cancer diagnosis. One woman had come to ACCESS with a lump in her breast. Despite numerous calls, the woman refused to get a mammogram. "Hiam comes to me and tells me she is not coming. Well she might have cancer and I needed to see that she goes. I said, how about if you go with her? Maybe she cannot speak good English. Maybe she does not have transportation to address these barriers, which women told us was why they weren't going. They didn't have cars or they didn't drive."

"Money also was an issue. The mammogram was $90 but that was too much then," before the expansion of insurance under the Affordable Care Act, he said. "I heard women saying, 'I can't do that. I don't have a spare $100.' I told Hiam you need to go with this woman, get her there, translate for her, and stay with her until she is done and you bring her back home. She still did not go."

Finally, Hammad asked Hamade to bring the woman in to see him. She told him, "I want my two daughters to get married," Hammad said. "After a second or so, I understood the dilemma."

"If she is diagnosed with cancer, she feared no one would come ask for her daughters' hands because of stigma. She'd rather die of cancer when no one knows she had it, rather than have her daughters know. And you know something? She didn't go. She refused and refused and refused. And I am sorry to say this woman didn't make it. That was culture and that is how culture impedes good health."

The incident motivated Hammad to do more. "I started going to Arabic cable TV and radio stations. I'd go to these little TV places and talk about the need for cancer screening among Arab women and men. I was attacked by Arab men. They said, 'How could you take our women away from their communities to be undressed in hospitals and health care systems we don't know?' Hiam, Ghada and I used to work so hard to overcome that."

ACCESS helps two thousand Arab women a year get mammograms, of whom forty-five to sixty are diagnosed with it.

"Now I see men coming with their wives for mammography at ACCESS. The women have surgery. They get on with their lives. So education can really lead to changes in people's health behavior. Education, assistance and steadfastness in doing the same mission can actually help people's attitudes and perceptions about health be changed. It was not easy. It was hard work. It still is very much needed."

17

Money and Insurance

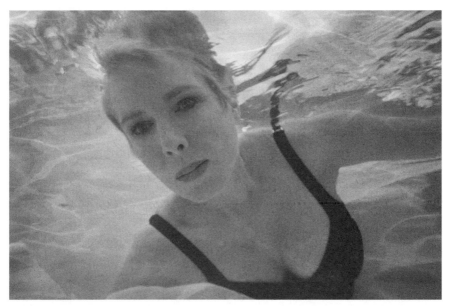

Molly MacDonald directs The Pink Fund, which helps pay nonmedical bills for women currently undergoing breast cancer treatment.

Molly MacDonald was in between jobs, supporting five children and paying $1,200 a month in health insurance when she was diagnosed with breast cancer in 2005.

Two lumpectomies and six weeks of daily radiation treatments delayed her career plans and ruined her household finances. She was the family's major breadwinner. Her husband is a piano technician whose income provides 30 percent of the household budget. When she couldn't work, their home in Beverly Hills, Michigan, went into foreclosure and they relied on a local food bank for a while.

Money even played into her choice of lumpectomy and radiation, she said. "I chose not to have reconstruction because of the additional cost of co-pays, the potential for infection and more treatment and more co-pays, as well as not being able to get a result I thought would please me," she said.

The experience left MacDonald, fifty-four at the time, thinking about other women like her. With women making up 47 percent of the American workforce, a breast cancer diagnosis can interrupt work, cause extended leaves from work, or result in job loss, she found.

"Half of all bankruptcies are caused by the cost of an illness or an illness that causes job loss," she said.

In 2005, she created The Pink Fund, a volunteer-led charity she incorporated a year later that has become one of the most established nonprofit organizations of its kind.

The Pink Fund provides as much as $3,000 to breast cancer patients currently in treatment for payment of nonmedical expenses, such as car insurance, mortgage payments, and utility bills. The organization's website, http://thepinkfund.org, explains how to apply for help and its eligibility guidelines. Though fund-raising has been challenging, the organization finished its most successful year ever in fiscal 2015, when it made $422,383.04 in bill payments for 363 breast cancer patients in forty-two states, a 51 percent increase from the last fiscal year, the group said.

It has distributed more than $1 million in the last eight years, raised from corporate and individual donations as well as fitness and health-related events. One of its most popular fund-raisers, held in seven large U.S. metropolitan areas, is a "Dancing with the Survivors®" event that teams professional dancers and breast cancer survivors or caregivers.

"The whole purpose of these events is to help women reclaim their sexuality and femininity," said MacDonald, an avid swimmer and athlete who participates in numerous health-related charity events. "Part of the challenge after surgery and reconstruction is, how do we reclaim intimacy with our partners? Dancing is a first step to getting back into the bedroom, where you feel safe."

One of the dancers at the fund's October 1, 2015, West Bloomfield, Michigan, event was Ty Weaver.

Weaver, forty-one, of Ypsilanti, Michigan, a widow with two children, eleven and fifteen, had to take a leave of absence from her church job when she was diagnosed with breast cancer in September 2014. She is the executive administrative assistant at the Strong Tower Ministries in Ypsilanti. She was out of work for the rest of 2014 and much of 2015, recovering from three surgeries: a lumpectomy that failed to get margins clear of cancer; a unilateral mastectomy with tissue-based reconstruction; and then a tune-up with a breast lift and construction of a new nipple and areola, in 2015. "I'm happy with it," she said.

She has gone for lengthy periods without health insurance since her husband died ten years ago, at age thirty-one, of a rare cancer.

Fortunately, through eligibility changes made in Medicaid guidelines through the Affordable Care Act, Weaver was able to get health insurance in 2014 because Michigan expanded its Medicaid program to cover more lower-income adults. She had been turned down for Medicaid coverage before the law, though her two children had health insurance through a state program.

The insurance covered nearly all of her expenses from a lumpectomy, then a unilateral mastectomy with tissue-based reconstruction in 2014.

"I didn't have a lot of out-of-pocket insurance expenses but I did have household expenses," she said. "When I had my surgery, I couldn't work. I'd be off six-to-eight weeks at a time. I wasn't allowed to drive for half that time. When I worked, that and Social Security benefits pretty much paid the bills. But when I couldn't work and I lost that income, it made it more difficult."

"A friend told me about the Pink Fund. I went online and found information and I submitted an application. A few months later, they contacted me and told me they could help pay my mortgage payments, gas and electric bills for two months. The bills amounted to about $2,000," she said.

"It helped a lot," Weaver said. "It took a lot of the weight off of me, worrying about where's the money going to come from."

⸺⸺⸺⸺◎⸺⸺⸺⸺

Alisa Savoretti, founder of My Hope Chest, a nonprofit organization that helps pay for reconstruction for uninsured and underinsured breast cancer survivors, always has far more applicants than she can help.

The Tampa-based organization works with breast cancer surgeons and plastic surgeons who agree to perform reconstruction at lower rates for uninsured or underinsured women. She always is looking for new surgeons to help. "We believe there are tens if not hundreds of thousands of breast cancer survivors who for one reason or another are unable to obtain their breast reconstruction," she said.

The nonprofit is able to help seven to ten of about one hundred women who apply each year, Savoretti said. The organization has helped about thirty women get breast reconstruction since 2010, after Savoretti reorganized it. It began as a fledgling charity in 2003.

"We receive most of our referrals from Susan G. Komen and the American Cancer Society," Savoretti said. "Many of these women want their

HEALTH INSURANCE AND BREAST CANCER SURGERY AND RECONSTRUCTION: WHAT'S COVERED

Since 1999, a federal law, the Women's Health and Cancer Rights Act (WHCRA), has required most health insurance companies that offer mastectomy coverage to also pay for reconstructive surgery after mastectomy. A health plan also must pay for reconstruction of the opposite noncancerous breast to give a more balanced look, as well as payments for breast prostheses and treatment of all physical complications of the mastectomy, including lymphedema, according to the Department of Labor, which administers the law.

The law, however, does not apply to Medicare or Medicaid programs, and some religious organizations and government health plans may be exempt. States also may have exemptions from the federal law that could affect benefits.

Two federal agencies, the U.S. Department of Labor and the U.S. Department Health and Human Services, oversee the law. Here's how to reach them:

Department of Labor

http://www.dol.gov/ebsa/Publications/whcra.html.

To order publications or request assistance from a benefits advisor, email askebsa.dol.gov or call 1-866-444-3272.

See also the Centers for Medicaid & Medicare Services, www.cms .gov.

STATE LAWS ON INSURANCE

The American Society of Plastic Surgeons has a state-by-state analysis of reconstruction coverage at: http://www.plasticsurgery .org/reconstructive-procedures/breast-reconstruction/breast-re construction-resources/state-laws-on-breast-reconstruction.

breasts restored but think they have nowhere to turn for help," Savoretti said. They lose their self-esteem and get depressed, she said. "It's an awful place for a woman to be who has already faced a life-or-death health issue."

The organization changed its eligibility criteria in 2015 to include payments to insured survivors with $2,500 to $6,000 in out-of-pocket costs.

Savoretti was thirty-eight and uninsured, taking a break from performing as a showgirl in Las Vegas when she was diagnosed with breast cancer. A local social service organization paid for her single mastectomy in March 2002, as well as eight rounds of chemotherapy. She called around hoping she'd find a local organization to pay for breast reconstruction but didn't find anything, she said. When she returned to her Vegas job five months after chemotherapy, she padded her costume and "no one knew," she said. She performed one-breasted for nearly two years until she underwent reconstruction with silicone implants.

"In hindsight, it worked out for me," she said about delayed reconstruction. "I wanted to deal with one thing at a time."

"I've had no problems, knock on wood," she said of her reconstruction. "I call my girls Zsa Zsa and Ava. Left is Zsa Zsa and the right is Ava. I'm grateful to have two breasts. My scar has faded a bit. My nipple healed flatter than when I started. But I don't think of those things. I don't have time to worry about it."

Savoretti worked side jobs as a nanny and bartender after she quit her career as a professional dancer. She said she refinanced her house three times while working hard to sustain her organization. "When the market flipped, I lost my home. That's why I came back to Florida," she said. She reorganized My Hope Chest in 2010 and in recent years has been developing a national board with several corporate sponsors, including Warner's Olga Bra, the Genie Bra, Dunkin' Donuts, and several Cadillac franchises.

In October 2014, a garment called "My Hope Chest Genie Bra" sold in 1,800 Walmart stores and earned $100,000, Savoretti said.

The organization holds several fund-raisers a year, but Savoretti acknowledged, "We're struggling to get to the next level." She wishes corporations and individuals will recognize her organization's "unique mission and redirect some donations to programs helping pay for reconstruction."

Savoretti said she is grateful for federal coverage of reconstruction for many insured women. "But people will still fall through the cracks of medical care. Just because there is a government mandate to have health care doesn't mean people have money to buy insurance," she said. "If people can't put food in their fridge and gas in their car, how can they buy government insurance? Are we going to throw people in jail because they can't pay their fines?"

"Our hope is to find a cure for breast cancer, sooner than later. Until that day happens, we need to help those who desire to find closure to cancer and make women whole again."

———————◆◆◆———————

In 2000, when Dr. Sandy Goldberg was diagnosed with breast cancer, she decided to take millions of people into the operating room for her quadrectomy surgery that removed a third of her breast.

"I thought, my viewers ought to know this," said Goldberg, sixty-nine, of Chicago, who is a health and nutrition contributor at NBC Chicago. "Talking about breast cancer in public wasn't taboo but it just wasn't done much."

The special report won an Emmy and got such terrific response that she created a cable TV program about cancer with an open phone line so experts could take questions from viewers.

One of the big issues, besides cancer treatment, was that some women couldn't afford to have a mammogram, let alone breast reconstruction. "I learned people felt they weren't worthy because they had no money and no insurance. That made me sick. I went home and cried, which I very seldom do. I told my husband and he said, 'What are you going to do about it, other than cry?' I said, 'Let's create a foundation.' The two of us at our kitchen table, with one $2,500 check, and we started A Silver Lining Foundation. It's based on the philosophy of my late mother. My parents were Russian Jewish immigrants who spoke Yiddish. Then, the father in the family wrote the checks and the mother explained what the bills were for. Mom would always say: 'We are all family. We have to help each other through the tough times.' In my mind, as we worked on the foundation, we always came back to that."

Since then, the foundation has helped more than nine thousand uninsured and underinsured women obtain mammograms and further diagnostic tests through its Buy a Mom a Mammogram® program. Its website, https://www.asilverliningfoundation.org, provides details. "We have women coming to us from Indiana, Michigan, Wisconsin and Ohio because they have no place to go." The programs mostly serve women in Chicago, Des Plaines, Evanston, Elgin, and Rockford. In 2014, it spent over $300,000 for those tests for about 1,200 women.

Thirteen partner hospitals provide access to screening and diagnostic mammograms as well as biopsies for women in the program. If diagnosed with breast cancer, they are not left hanging, she said. "All our partner hospitals agreed on the front end to assure that any women with breast cancer won't be told, 'have a nice day.'" Goldberg said. The hospitals also have patient navigators who enroll women into the federally and state-funded programs to gain access to surgery and treatment.

Guy Medaglia, president and chief executive officer of St. Anthony Hospital, in Chicago, said the foundation's help has been invaluable. "By partnering with A Silver Lining Foundation, we have increased access to much-needed screening and diagnostic mammography services for women who otherwise do not have access to such care," Medaglia said. "The foundation's programs allow us to educate and screen more patients before it is too late."

While the Affordable Care Act of 2010 has helped women get screening for mammograms, many gaps remain, Goldberg said.

"For those individuals who manage to qualify for Medicaid, at least have something they didn't have before," she said. "What we are seeing are enormous gaps in the system, including Medicaid. For example, you don't qualify for ACA if you don't have a checking account. But 25 percent of the American public does not have a checking account. This is the kind of stuff we deal with all the time. If you work and by some miracle you are given a small raise that can kick you out of Medicaid. You have no idea what that means to an individual. You can buy the insurance but can you afford the copays and the deductibles? Then of course if you are under 40 and need testing, that's too bad. If you don't meet the income guidelines or can't afford the coverage, it's good luck to you." She hopes to expand the reach of the foundation to other cities.

She still hears too many stories of women delaying tests to find breast cancer. "One woman we saw recently had a large lump that clearly was there for a while. She told the foundation she delayed getting tested because she said, 'I have to feed my kids.'"

"It makes me sick. That's what drives me."

18

Clothing and Breast Forms

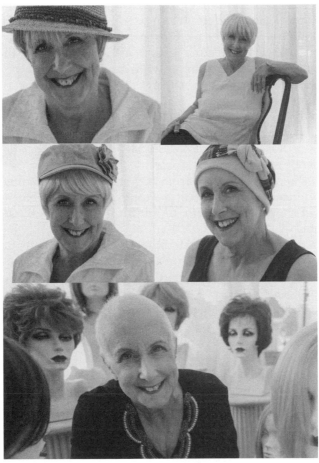

Dr. Linda Jo Johnson saw a certified mastectomy fitter when she was diagnosed with breast cancer so she'd have the right things she needed after surgery

Dr. Linda Jo Johnson knew it was time for the trip she had avoided.

Her hair was falling out in large clumps from chemotherapy, and she had to face the obvious. She needed a wig.

Later she would need a post-surgery bra after her lumpectomy, and she had questions of all sorts about how she'd look after the operation and what she might need to look stylish and pretty.

She and her husband, Bob, headed to Susan's Special Needs, a Pleasant Ridge, Michigan, mastectomy boutique owned by Susan Thomas, a certified mastectomy fitter, breast cancer survivor, and oncology nurse.

Certified fitters such as Thomas are experts who know breast forms and other mastectomy products the way plastic surgeons know breast implants.

To gain certification, fitters must spend at least five hundred hours fitting women for breast forms, bras, compression garments, and other post-surgery and cancer treatment supplies. The websites of the Board of Certification/Accreditation, http://www.bocusa.org, and the American Board for Certification, www.abcop.org, help women find certified mastectomy fitters in their areas.

Certified fitters can be employed by large medical device firms, by hospitals, by private health care specialists, or through independent shops such as Susan's Special Needs. Medicare and other health plans restrict members to buying durable medical equipment, the term for surgery bras and breast forms, from companies designated by Medicare or the insurance company as contractors. Women purchasing items at independent shops may have to submit forms to be reimbursed by their health plans.

Most health plans, as well as Medicare, help pay for many mastectomy products, such as a post-surgery bra and one breast form every two years, Thomas said. Women should expect to pay their usual deductibles and other out-of-pocket expenses for these products, she said.

Three to six weeks after surgery, when the breast has completely healed, most women are ready to wear a bra, and if desired, a breast form. Bras should not be worn if there is tenderness or any swelling or breakdown in the skin.

Breast forms come in dozens of types, shapes, and materials. There are full forms for mastectomy patients and smaller fillers for women to fill in gaps in their breast after a lumpectomy. They may be made of silicone, polyurethane foam, or cloth. Foam and cloth types are lighter, cooler, and have advantages for leisure and sleep, but they may ride up or move when women wear them for dress-up, she said.

Silicone breast forms come in various weights, in everyday, sportswear, sleep, and swim models. Some forms are filled with microbeads to aid in quick drying. Lightweight, perspiration-resistant silicone forms address long-time problems, from perspiration to shifting and dislodgement outside of clothing.

American Breast Care, one large manufacturer, has a Diamond breast form that advertises how it helps a woman "stay cooler; reduce perspiration; minimize breast form shifting; and experience maximum comfort." It comes in a pink suede travel case.

There are more products, too, for larger women, but women who have bust measurements beyond a DDD cup "have a difficult time," Thomas said. "There have not been many companies that make bras for these women. They have a difficult time particularly if they had unilateral surgery. The breast forms are heavy. That's where I learned how to customize bras to give the forms more support."

Other forms attach to the chest wall with a medical-grade adhesive. They can be worn with a non-mastectomy bra or without a bra. "They take weight off the shoulders," Thomas said. "Whether a woman can wear one requires an assessment. It depends on the typography of the chest wall, whether it's flat, where there are hills and valleys, and it also depends on the size of the tumor and the kind of surgery doctors do."

An appointment with a certified fitter should begin with a complete assessment and physical, Thomas explained. "I look at chest walls. I'm looking at the size and shape of the existing breast as well as the breast form. If you go to someone with no experience or you buy breast forms out of a catalog, you as a patient don't know what you need. And when you wear it it is uncomfortable."

Thomas, who had a unilateral mastectomy without reconstruction in 1992, dispenses a range of advice and products. Some women, and some couples, come to see the real deal. It's a kind of show-and-tell she doesn't advertise.

"I undress in front of people I don't know," Thomas said. "I show women and their husbands my mastectomy scars. If people see my scar, they say, 'OK, I can do that. It's not so bad.'" She also frequently demonstrates how she can quickly insert a breast form into the pocket of her mastectomy bra.

Thomas works with tailors who can customize bras and other items. She said that about 20 percent of her customers need custom tailoring. "As a fitter, I find what I need to do to tailor a bra so it fits. Whatever I need to customize that bra, that's what we do here. Bilateral patients particularly need to be sure their bras fit perfectly. They don't have something to anchor the bra. If the bra choice is wrong, it rides up and then their breast forms are up underneath their chin. I'm a perfectionist in terms of that." A common question she's asked: "Do I have to wear it all the time? Women call and say, 'Susan, my breast form is too heavy.' I ask, 'How often are you wearing it?' 'Oh, only to church on Sundays.'

Well, if you are wearing it once a week, it's going to feel like a new pair of shoes every time you put it on. You have to wear it every day so your brain catches up with your body's perception of how you look and how you feel in a bra."

A widely unacknowledged problem she sees are women whose breasts shrink years after radiation. "It happens down the road," Thomas said. These women can be evaluated for a pocketed bra and partial breast form, she said.

Fitters like Thomas can be particularly helpful to women like Johnson, who has chest tenderness and pain from lymphedema she developed after radiation and an axillary lymph node dissection that removed eight nodes. She keeps it at bay with massage exercises she learned in physical therapy and a compression sleeve she wears when she flies. She sometimes wears a thick compression bandage over her chest. "She taught me how to do it," Johnson said of her lymphedema specialist, Cynthia Tan, with the Beaumont Health system in Royal Oak, Michigan.

Johnson's insurance did not cover the compression bra or sleeve she purchased to reduce lymphedema. She considers these and other clothing investments worthwhile because her lymphedema has lessened significantly.

Her hair has grown back, curlier than before. She fondly remembers the day she picked up her first wig at Susan's.

"My husband drove me to Susan's, went to the market to get some groceries and came back to get me," she said. She recalled how Susan's husband, Dave Thomas, coaxed Thompson's husband, Bob, into the store "for the big reveal of me with my new wig, so we waited until he parked and then invited him in (I think by phone). It was a happy day for all of us."

19

Doctor Selection Issues

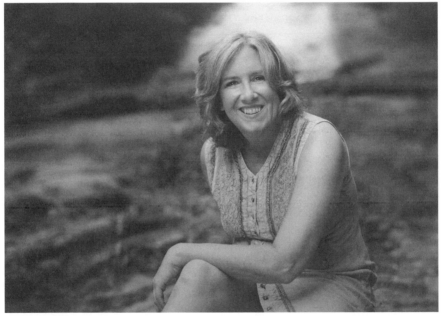

Belinda Cox didn't get her first choice of a plastic surgeon. Now she wonders if she should have gone to someone else.

Belinda Cox didn't get to pick the plastic surgeon who performed her breast cancer reconstruction.

Her insurance company did.

She and her breast surgeon asked her insurance company to let her see another doctor in the area, who is not part of the plan's network, but the company turned down her appeal.

She waited more than two years for reconstruction, hoping her company would switch insurance plans, then went ahead with the surgery.

Today she has regrets. Sometimes, she wonders whether she ever would have had reconstruction at all if she had done more research.

"In retrospect, I would have had them both taken off and I would not have opted for reconstruction," said Cox, forty-seven, of Asheville, North Carolina. "I would have gotten me a nice tattoo."

Finding the right doctor and medical team can be a challenge for women facing breast cancer surgery.

FINDING A BOARD-CERTIFIED DOCTOR

These resources provide help finding board-certified doctors and talking to them.

- National Cancer Institute: www.cancer.gov/about-cancer/ coping/adjusting-to-cancer/talk-with-doctors
- American Society of Clinical Oncology, www.cancer.net/ cancer-types/breast-cancer/questions-ask-doctor
- American Society of Plastic Surgeons, www1.plasticsurgery .org/find_a_surgeon
- American Board of Plastic Surgery, www.certificationmatters .org/is-your-doctor-board-certified.aspx
- American Society for Reconstructive Microsurgery, www.mi crosurg.org/physicians/search/

Health insurance plans limit a woman's choice of both her physicians and hospital. Going out of network, as Cox wanted, costs more, typically 25 percent of a bill, and may force many women to stay within their health network.

What doctor a woman gets and the type of reconstruction she may choose also largely depend on where a woman lives. Most plastic surgeons practice in urban areas, and some states still don't have many microvascular experts who routinely perform breast reconstruction with a woman's own tissue and blood vessels.

Practice patterns within a hospital also dictate doctor referrals that breast surgeons make to patients about plastic surgeons. Most breast surgeons operate with one or two preferred plastic surgeons, and those doctors by far perform implant-based breast reconstruction.

"Breast surgeons have a lot of impact on a patient's decision making," said Dr. Kongrit Chaiyasate, a microvascular plastic surgeon in Royal Oak, Michigan, with the Beaumont Health system. "They refer patients to plastic surgeons they trust, like their old buddy from medical school. All he does is implants. Women aren't told about all the options available."

Women, for example, often are told that tissue-based breast reconstruction is not a good option for those who have had radiation, Chaiyasate said. While more challenging, women who have had radiation still achieve good results, he said. "Plastic surgeons should not make comments to discourage patients about procedures they do not do," he said.

The problem has led some states such as New York to pass laws requiring women to be informed of their reconstruction choices. There also are legislative efforts to do the same nationally.

What follows are some examples that explain the different ways that women get their breast cancer surgery teams and their insights about handling varied issues and problems along the way. The chapter also provides resources for finding a good doctor.

———————◦«◉»◦———————

Belinda Cox remembers her diagnosis with stage 2 ductal breast cancer as "bang, bang, bang."

She found the lump herself March 27, 2012, and within the month she underwent a unilateral skin-sparing mastectomy without reconstruction.

Cox hoped to move quickly to have breast reconstruction, but her insurance posed a major obstacle. The plastic surgeon her breast surgeon recommended most was not covered by her health insurance. Her health plan only would allow her to see another plastic surgeon whom the breast surgeon said "would not be my first choice," Cox recalled. "So I did not have the reconstruction done right away."

She waited more than two-and-a-half years, hoping the environmental company where she worked as an archeologist would change health plans, as it did before. "So we waited and waited." Finally, her surgeon suggested she consider reconstruction with the doctor in her plan because he had done a good job on another one of her other patients.

"It really was my doctor's recommendation," Cox explained. "Before my breast doctor suggested I go back, I was happy to live with it just the way it was," she said. "I had decided I didn't want to do it. She said, 'You will look really good. I can refer you.' I said, If you are ok with it, I'm ok with it."

Cox is a lesbian with plans to marry her long-time partner, Cat, in 2015. She had the same motivations most women do who want breast reconstruction. "I'm a woman first," Cox said. "That is part of being a woman. I love my breasts."

When she met with the plastic surgeon she had delayed seeing, he chided her for waiting so long for reconstruction, she said.

She said he asked her, "'Why didn't you have this done?' I didn't want to tell him I didn't want him so I told him I had enough of surgery. He said, 'Oh, that's a bad phrase around here. There's never too much surgery.'"

They discussed her procedure, and he showed her dozens of before and after photos of patients he had reconstructed. They looked good, better than what she had expected. She decided to go ahead. She had no interest in reconstruction with her own tissue. "Too many scars. That scared me more. I never considered that."

In December 2014, she had unilateral breast reconstruction with a silicone implant.

She found the expander phase of the procedure "extremely painful," and she rued her decision to have reconstruction but decided she had invested so much time in it, she'd see it through.

She returned to the doctor in May 2015 for nipple reconstruction and a liposuction-like procedure to transfer tummy fat to her breast to shape and hold the implant better. She and her medical oncologist agreed that what she got wasn't a breast lift. The plastic surgeon had just moved her nipple and stretched the areola. Her breasts still didn't match. "It was exactly the same, except my nipple is higher and surrounded by a very large areola," Cox said.

"I am really unhappy. It's scarred. I didn't realize it was going to involve cutting the entire nipple. They went under and around the nipple and made what he called a lollipop cut. The skin is supposed to be pinched together, which causes the breast to move up."

She described her breasts as "Frankenboobs," a common reference others also make about breasts reconstructed with implants. "This one didn't get a mastopexy so it looks a lot the same except it has a lot more scars. The nipple and areola are a third of the entire breast. It's huge. It's never going to be the cute little thing it was. The other one is still really bruised from the nipple construction he did and the painful liposuction he performed beneath my belly button."

Looking back, Cox wishes she had listened to her inner doubts, done more research, and asked more questions, particularly about how a procedure is done and what the recovery would be like.

She also understands that paying more money on her own might have gotten her a doctor she was happier with. She is left to wonder. She asked, "If I had chosen to go out of network and paid a lot more money, and I had seen the other doctor the breast surgeon recommended, would I have had a skin-sparing mastectomy with better results?"

She urged other women to think carefully about their doctor choices because they will live with the results of their work for years to come.

————————◆————————

Trish Gallagher did exhaustive research when she was diagnosed in January 2008 with ductal carcinoma in situ, an early-stage breast cancer, but hers had aggressive cells described as having microinvasion to nearby tissue.

Gallagher, fifty-eight, was eligible for either a lumpectomy and radiation or mastectomy. She felt pressured to pick lumpectomy, which she found irritating.

"I interviewed five breast surgeons in New York City, each at the top of their game," said Gallagher, PhD, an assistant clinical professor of medical psychology at Columbia University, College of Physicians and Surgeons and a clinical psychologist at New York Presbyterian Hospital/Columbia Medical Center, in New York.

"Nobody, nobody told me that a bilateral mastectomy would be the best move for me," she said. "I had things said to me like, 'Don't you want to hold on to your breasts a little longer?' I said, 'Hello, the breasts are what could kill me. I think not."

"I will never forget an interview with the head of breast surgery" at one New York hospital, she said. "I sat with a friend and physician on one side and my husband on the other, and I said, 'Excuse me. You are telling me to get a lumpectomy. There's a 50% chance of invasive recurrence in 20 years. You see these people sitting next to me? They are my support system. Where are they going to be in 20 years and how will I feel in 20 years? Lumpectomy. I think not.' I went back to work and called my breast surgeon and said, 'Here's what I want you to do and here's how I want you to do it.'"

Gallagher, a mother of two boys, preferred not to take a chance. She had a double mastectomy with silicone breast reconstruction. Her husband went as far as telling her, "I think you're making a big mistake," she said.

Though she felt she made the right choice, she found the preoperative surgical markings unnerving and her recovery worse than what she expected, she said.

"I don't know if it was just my experience," she said, "but the way mastectomies are done is horrible. Not because of the procedure, which has advanced greatly, but because there is a time from when you walk up the ramp to the surgeon's office, you are marked with a pen the way cattle is probably marked for butchering."

"I also was not prepared for how I would look after surgery and not just waking up with what delightfully are called breast mounds. I was not prepared for the extent of the bruising. I looked like I was hit by a bus. I looked at myself and I just screamed. I spent six weeks recovering. Nobody but nobody prepared me for the neuropathic pain I would endure as the nerve cells regenerated in my breast," she said. "I tried at least three different pain meds and nothing touched that pain. There is no feeling like nerve cells regenerating. It is excruciating and nobody talks about it. The other thing no one prepared me about is that reconstruction is a multi-step, many-year process. It doesn't happen in one shot if you want it done correctly."

Gallagher recommends thoroughly checking out plastic surgeons to find out which type of reconstruction operations they perform the most and what their success is with nipple reconstruction. "The person who does the implants is not necessarily the person who is gifted at nipple reconstruction," she said. "You have to be really careful and surgeon shop."

Gallagher expects she will have another revision. "My left boob looked fabulous. My right boob looked like it hadn't had an implant after a few months. I have one breast now that is shorter in length than the other breast and kind of squared off. I'm currently looking at a third revision and I'm disappointed."

Gallagher made a list of recommendations for others facing surgery.

- Does the doctor listen well? "First of all they have to listen to you and be able to take direction."
- Bring your doctor pictures of your breasts. "I'd advise any woman facing a mastectomy to take pictures of her breasts and bring them everywhere, and say, 'Guys, this is what I want you to recreate. Can you do it? I'd like a breast that looks like my old breast, thank you.'"
- Understand that reconstruction "is a multistep process. It will take years. No one will tell you this but it will take years."
- "Be patient and be determined to get what you want. Breasts are incredibly important to us all. They are our sexuality."
- Check out state doctor records on disciplinary actions.
- Ask to speak with patients the doctor has treated.

———=◉=———

Julie Morang grew up in metro Detroit, where people talk about closely inspecting and test driving a car before buying one.

She went about finding a doctor the same way after her diagnosis in 2006 at age fifty-two with a stage 2 lobular breast cancer. The tumor had spread to four lymph nodes, which worried her. A single mother, her daughter, now grown, was thirteen at the time.

"I wasn't going to have a major procedure done without first touching, feeling and kicking the tires," said Morang, a small business owner who lives in Grosse Pointe Park, Michigan. "You have to pick and choose carefully. Get a second opinion. You have to be your own patient advocate or you'll fall through the cracks, as you would with any medical procedure."

Over three years of treatment, Morang had more than a dozen medical procedures and treatments, including three lumpectomies, chemotherapy, radiation, and a bilateral mastectomy with silicone breast reconstruction.

From the beginning, she took time to find the right doctors. She interviewed several plastic surgeons before picking one she liked. She talked to women who had reconstruction to see their results firsthand, not just from a photo. And when she still had cancer after two lumpectomies, she went to the University of Michigan for a second opinion that changed the course of her treatment for the better, she said.

U-M had told her that because she still had traces of cancer after two lumpectomies, she would need more surgery and chemotherapy. U-M used a standard that required two millimeters of clean margins around a tumor as a guide to additional surgery; St. John at the time had a standard of one millimeter.

"The University of Michigan opinion from Dr. Daniel Hayes was very critical to everything," Morang said. "Had I not gotten that second opinion from U-M, I would have walked away from two lumpectomies and still had cancer. And I never would have had a mastectomy."

After four months of chemotherapy and a third lumpectomy, "everybody was in total shock there was still cancer, me, most of all," she said. "At that point, I said, 'I don't want to trust another lumpectomy or more chemo.' I already had gone through four months of chemo. At that point, I was done debating between bilateral versus single mastectomy. Radiation was to come."

She credits her breast surgeon with the St. John Health Providence health system in metro Detroit for her willingness to accept a slightly different course of treatment prescribed for Morang at U-M. "She was very gracious about it."

Morang had been with the surgeon from the beginning. She gave Morang one plastic surgeon's name, and Morang easily found two others through women who had breast reconstruction, lived near her, and were willing to talk about it.

The first plastic surgeon "I didn't like at all," Morang said. "He was brusque and aloof." The second doctor did many types of plastic surgery rather than specializing mostly in breast surgery, which was not what she wanted. The third plastic surgeon "was polite and answered all my questions," so she went with him. She asked the doctor for patients willing to talk about their surgery. Then she went and talked to a few in person.

"Women were extremely helpful," she recalled. "Many let me touch and feel their breasts to see what their implants looked like and felt like. One neighbor had gone through a double mastectomy. She let me see her breasts. That kind of pushed me, to see how you have breasts that match with a double mastectomy."

"I wanted to feel what silicone felt like," Morang said. "It gave me the courage to go through it." Her openness is shared by many breast cancer survivors, who say they often allow others, including strangers, to see what a reconstructed breast or a mastectomy or lumpectomy scar looks like.

Initially, Morang did not want a mastectomy. But when she decided on a mastectomy, everyone seemed to encourage her to do it. "Everyone says, 'Oh get it done,'" she said. "And you have actresses like Angelina Jolie getting it done. She's absolutely gorgeous. Look at me. I had a double mastectomy. I'm still absolutely gorgeous. She is. But you don't see the pain she went through."

"I am glad actresses are out there now saying that they had it done but no one is talking about the pain involved. I wish they would. Women may opt not to do the plastic surgery. I'd like to see an actress say, no, I'm not going to have breast implants."

Morang, who had a mother who had breast cancer and an aunt who died of it at age fifty-five, had genetic tests to see if she carried a mutation that raised her risk of breast and ovarian cancer.

"The test came back negative for me. I felt good for that result, at least for my daughter."

She chose silicone implant reconstruction, primarily because she finds tissue-based reconstruction brutal on a woman's body.

"In terms of what's good for your body, no surgery would be good for your body," said Morang. "But I'm young and I want my clothes to fit properly. So I went with silicone. Water didn't have the same feel. This is only supposed to last for about 10 years. I'll be due about 2017. I had expanders put in. What no one tells any woman is how painful everything is. There's so much going on. One of my best friends is a nurse in Chicago. She went through the same procedures I did. She said she's sorry she put the implants in, she's been in so much pain from that."

"Expanders feel like having an elephant put on your chest. You can't breathe. It doesn't subside. When you sleep at night, your chest feels so tight, so heavy. In my case, they had to fill the expanders three times as fast because they wanted me to get to the radiation phase. The radiation was no cakewalk either. I am fair-skinned and burn easily. Radiation burned me to a crisp."

It took several procedures to get Morang's breasts to match. "They're fine," Morang said. "They are not like my regular breasts were. They are a sportier version. I was always large-breasted. As a young girl, I felt uncomfortable with that. Now I don't always have to wear a bra. The only time I wear a bra now is when I wear a dress and I want a better shape."

When she talks to other women with breast cancer, answering their questions and sometimes even showing her reconstruction results, as other women did for her, Morang emphasizes finding the right doctors.

"Through all of it, the scariest part was getting the right doctors and surgeons, a team," she said. "That's where you have to be your own patient advocate and constantly be seeking knowledge about methods of treatment."

━━━━◦«◉»◦━━━━

Dr. Marla Rowe Gorosh is an expert in patient and physician communication in the Detroit-based Henry Ford Healthcare System's Department of Family Medicine.

She has worked with consumer groups to teach how to prepare for a doctor visit, and she has taught classes to doctors on how to deliver bad news.

She also is a breast cancer survivor who underwent a lumpectomy at age thirty-eight, with radiation and chemotherapy.

Preparation for the first visit with a doctor is important, but "don't overload yourself," she said. "If you are the kind of person who wants to gather all the information first, I'd say go to the Internet but find a reputable website." Write your questions down, she advised.

For the visit, "Bring somebody so they can be your ears and ask the questions you have brought," she said. "Bring a tape recorder and ask if you can record it so you can go back to it."

"The kinds of questions to ask are the universal questions: 'What's my life going to look like in the next year? How often will I be seen?' Women always ask, 'Will I need surgery again? How often do you have to go back in and re-excise the lesion because you don't have clear margins? How many infections do you have post op? Will I need a drain? Will I need a port?'"

If a woman isn't comfortable with the responses, she should look elsewhere, Gorosh said. "There is a winning over, on the part of a patient and the physician. Patients walk away because they don't feel doctors addressed the needs for their visit."

She teaches physicians a set of patient communications skills, shortened to an acronym, PEARLS, that is used to address emotions and provide empathic statements.

It was developed by the American Academy on Communications in Healthcare to provide health care workers with empathic statements they could use with patients. The concepts and some examples she gave are:

"P is for Partnership statements. It's so good you are here today. We're going to work on this with you. I've got to make sure you will go away feeling satisfied and that all your questions have been answered. Make 3–4–5 of those kinds of partnership statements."

"E is for emotion. If someone is hyped up or anxious, you name it. I can see this is really a tough time for you."

"Apologize. I am so sorry this is set up this way. I'm so sorry you have to be here."

"Respect. No wonder you are so strong. You've lived through so much. I give you so much credit for coming in, despite how you are feeling. You've done beautifully. Thank you for being so cooperative."

"L is for legitimatization: anyone would feel this way."

"S is silence. Silence has its own strength."

20

Previvors

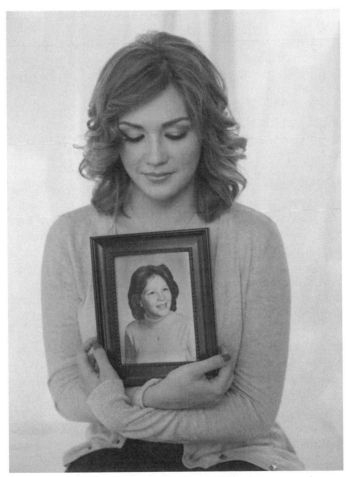

Kelly Rothe is one of the youngest American women to have a preventive double mastectomy. She was twenty. She is holding a photo of her mother, who died of breast cancer when Kelly was nine.

At twenty, she was believed to be one of the youngest American women ever known to get a preventive mastectomy.

Kelly Rothe, a college junior at the time, was strong and confident explaining how she came to her decision. She lives with purpose, sharing her story so other young women confronted with similar decisions will understand how she came to her choices. A tattoo on her back, next to a pink ribbon, carries a lifelong directive: "To whom much is given, much is expected."

"Hi. I'm Kelly Rothe. I'm 20. I will be 21 in August," she said at a May 8, 2014, media briefing at Beaumont Hospital, Royal Oak, Michigan, where she had her preventive bilateral mastectomy with silicone implant reconstruction.

"On Friday, I'm having a double mastectomy because I have the BRCA1 gene. Right now I have an 87% risk I will get breast cancer in the next 20 years. To me the choice was easy. Growing up, I watched my mother go through breast cancer and I watched what it did to my family. I wouldn't want to do that to my kids. So this is a time in my life when I can take some time off of school and really allow myself to recover the way I want to and the way that's healthiest for me."

In 1994, BRCA1 was the first gene identified as a cause of breast and ovarian cancer when it is mutated or changed; BRCA2 was found the next year. Both are called susceptibility genes. Neither causes cancer.

Mutations in these genes suggest a person's greater chance of having cancer. These tumors usually aren't considered more aggressive or deadlier, unless a woman is diagnosed with breast cancer at a young age. Women with these mutations sometimes call themselves previvors.

Kelly was nine, with twin younger siblings, when her mother died. "For me the decision was easy," said Rothe, who has acquired some national media attention for her story, including a leading role in a Hollywood documentary about hereditary breast cancer in men and women.

"It came right after I got the results of my genetic test results. They tell you the recommended age to do this is 30. I knew I wouldn't wait that long. I thought I'd at least be 25 or 26. It was just a matter of doctor's approval and the time in my life." Rothe said she "wouldn't say I'm doing this in honor of my mom. I'm doing this completely on my own. It was my decision definitely."

Preventive surgeries sought by women without cancer but at high risk of it are one of the biggest, most stunning developments in breast reconstruction of the last decade.

Twenty years ago, few would fathom that a college junior like Rothe would voluntarily undergo surgery to remove her breasts because she had a high risk of breast and ovarian cancer.

WHAT'S THE ORIGIN OF THE WORD *PREVIVOR*?

Sue Friedman, a Florida veterinarian, said she coined the term around 2008 after realizing that women with a hereditary risk of breast and ovarian cancer needed a word to describe them. She had started a nonprofit, Facing Our Risk Collectively Empowered (FORCE), a decade earlier, only to find women with gene mutations felt excluded in breast cancer circles.

"The medical community was using the term *unaffected carrier*," recalled Friedman, a breast cancer survivor and BRCA2 carrier. "You carried a gene mutation but you were unaffected by the disease." Unaffected hardly seemed to be the case, she said. "As I started meeting more women with the genetic mutation and I saw how they approached the idea of support, kind of apologetically, I thought, we need to unite this community. One of our board members said on our message board, I need a label. I lost my mom to cancer. I lost my breasts to cancer. I lost my fertility to cancer. But I don't have cancer. What am I? So we actually put out a request through our community for a call for terms. There were some light-hearted ones. At the end of the day, I came up with the term, a pre-vivor with a predisposition to cancer. Everyone didn't love it. There was some high-profile criticism of the term. It was a way to provide a label to unite a community of stakeholders who really were not in a place at the table." Not long afterward, Friedman was delighted to read that *Time* magazine chose the word as one of the ten best new words of the year.

As genetic testing improved, public interest in these prophylactic procedures increased. But things really changed in 2013 when actress Angelina Jolie publicly announced she has undergone such preventive procedures.

So many women sought genetic counseling and preventive surgeries afterward that top cancer centers called it the Angelina effect. "I've even had people use the terminology, I want to be tested for the Angelina gene, or they'll say, I have the Angelina thing going on in my family," said Dr. Dana Zakalik, director of cancer genetics at Beaumont, who helped test and advise Rothe about the implications of having a BRCA gene defect.[1]

Women who seek preventive surgeries undergo the operations at the risk of harming their health to get as much as a 90 percent reduction in their risk of breast cancer and 50 percent of ovarian cancer.

But there are clear tradeoffs to risk-reduction surgeries. A healthy woman undergoing preventive surgery can develop infections, symmetry, and other problems that may need months of revisions.

Women who undergo implant reconstruction lose sensation in their breasts, as do many who have tissue-based methods. Surgical removal of the ovaries also causes women to abruptly enter menopause that triggers mood swings, hot flashes, and loss of sexual drive. Some women take estrogen-based hormone therapies to enhance their sex lives, though there is controversy about whether women at risk of breast cancer should take any estrogen therapy.

For those and other reasons, cancer centers won't test women for breast or ovarian cancer until they are eighteen.

"The decision to have a prophylactic mastectomy is very individual and personalized," said Rothe's breast surgeon, Dr. Nayana Dekhne, at the press briefing. "Kelly chose to do this at 20. But there are no guidelines that suggest these things be done at a certain age."

Rothe was nineteen when she first met Dekhne. She had to convince her she was mature enough to know what she was doing.

"When I first saw Kelly, I said, 'Kelly I'm not doing this. I don't think you should go through this. We should continue to follow you.' I was going over her family history and when I saw a 20-year-old on my schedule of appointments, I said to my staff, if you are booking 20-year-olds seeking mastectomies, you are wasting my time. They said, 'Why don't you go in and see who she is.' After I talked to her, I was convinced she had made her decision."

Rothe remembered Dekhne saying, "Kelly, I don't know why you are here." The teenager boldly responded, "Are you willing to listen?"

Rothe recounted her family history and won the doctor over. "It was just the way I spoke," Rothe said. "I was very certain. I still am very certain of my decision."

≈《◉》≈

In December 2010, Karen Lazarovitz, forty-one, of Montreal, began the BRCA Sisterhood, the largest private hereditary breast and ovarian cancer group on Facebook. It connects women with hereditary risks with resources, support, and advice and love from others dealing with similar issues, Lazarovitz said. It is a closed page that requires authorization by the site's administrators to post comments.

What she does not share, at least not initially, is how a woman with healthy breasts developed serious problems after a preventive double mastectomy with silicone implant reconstruction.

It took five procedures over three years to get the breasts she now has and likes.

"I have no regrets about my decision," said Lazarovitz, a mother of two elementary schoolchildren who works in sales and purchasing for a computer company. "Whatever happened in my story, I wouldn't do differently. But I did have complications. I wasn't prepared. I expected one surgery and that was that."

Lazarovitz has a BRCA2 mutation, one of the genetic deletions first identified in Ashkenazi Jews like her. "I'm a typical 1 in 40 Ashkenazi Jew who has this Jewish mutation. I have one of the DNA Ashkenazi founder mutations. There's three of them. My mutation is 6174 delT," citing the precise location of the chromosomal rearrangement.

Deciding to have a total hysterectomy was an easy decision, she said. "We already were fortunate enough to have children, a boy and a girl. We were very content with our family so it wasn't a huge mind-alternating decision for me. I found out about this when my family already was complete."

She had a minimally invasive, robotic hysterectomy on February 10, 2012, at Montreal Jewish General Hospital. "As soon as I healed from hysterectomy, I started preparing for my mastectomy," she said.

Within two months, she completed her plan with a preventive double mastectomy with tissue expanders for six months and then silicone implant reconstruction. What she hoped would be a quick operation to help her regain her well-being and body image became a three-year ordeal to get her breasts fixed.

In the months after her plastic surgeon swapped her saline expanders for silicone implants, her implants shifted and started moving south. The pain was so bad she took seven months off work.

"My right implant slipped out of the pocket in my chest and it started migrating lower," she said. "I don't blame the plastic surgeon for this. I am not angry. Surgeons are not God. Nobody heals the same. Basically what happened is my implant slipped. I started getting pain in my rib cage. I went back in right away. It's hard to explain when an implant is moving how terribly painful it can be."

The doctor told her to give her chest time to heal and for the implants to settle in. "Six months later, he brought me back in and did a little stitching. He did a little bit of fat-grafting injections which he said was going to help with the pain issues. I was quite sore. It looked a little better but I could see things didn't feel right. Nothing felt perfect."

"About six months later, I wasn't feeling good. The implant slipped again. He went back in and they stitched it in. After that, I came home and I had a violent reaction to the anesthesia and I was vomiting the whole night. I'm convinced that with all that vomiting and retching, it reopened the incision. They brought me back to the hospital. About two months after that, my implant slipped again and dropped an inch lower than the other one. Then I was in terrible pain, in my arm, my shoulder blade, my rib cage. I started talking to my husband. I told him, 'I need a new surgeon.'"

"You get stuck in that loophole of that surgeon who is treating you. You feel like you are going behind his back because you don't want to step on anyone's toes. Sometimes plastic surgeons don't like referrals. So for a year, I was going through this pain. They put me on Lyrica, because I had all this pain and I had a hard time functioning."

"And by then the breast with the affected implant was two inches lower than the other side. I had pain, plus I was embarrassed. I didn't look right. I started doing research. I had created this online network, so I knew about the Alloderm and other options that my surgeon wasn't interested in. He said, 'I don't do that. It's not necessary.' The doctor actually said, 'They don't look that bad. Your own breasts aren't perfect. If you find it that painful you always can take the implant out.' I said to him, 'You want to leave me breast-less? That's not going to happen.'"

"I said to him in tears, 'If your daughter came to you like this, would you help her?'"

"I had already started looking for a different doctor. It was during that time my husband had this epiphany. He's quiet and he doesn't get involved unless he feels he needs to. He actually said, 'You better give my wife a referral to someone who will fix her.' He was so angry. During that time I started calling other surgeons."

Finally, she was able to get in to see Dr. Karl Schwarz, a Montreal plastic surgeon, and she laid out her story.

"He listened to what I had to say. I said, 'I've created this community of support with over 5,000 women. I know a lot more than the standard person about these procedures. If you can't do what I want, that's OK. Just tell me you can't and I'll go speak with a doctor who can.' I came in as a business-minded patient, not as a poor-me patient, whom doctors don't always respond to as well."

"He didn't want to do surgery right away. Everything was pulling. He wanted to put me on pain pills for four months to trick my body that the pain was going away. He wanted to change the nerve pain."

Then in a procedure on March 4, 2012, "he started from scratch and he took out everything that the other doctor did. This was two years later. He used textured implants, which he said he preferred because they adhere better to your skin. He used a high-profile teardrop-shaped implant because he said it looked more realistic. He stitched me differently and used Alloderm as a sling under the implant for extra support. It probably was the most painful surgery I had of all five of them, besides the mastectomy."

Still, the surgery gave her a big sense of relief, almost immediately, she said.

"It was worth all the pain. I would have done it over a million times. I just wish I had known all the things that could have happened. I'm not talking about the issues on the form surgeons make you sign. I'm talking about real, everyday stories. I just wish I would have mentally known it would have been a longer haul."

―――――⟪◉⟫―――――

Lazarovitz likes her results. "I think they look pretty good. I think I look really good in a shirt. You'd never know I had implants. I think because I've had so many complications, I've become very removed from my breasts. When I look at them in the mirror, they look pretty good. My right side always is a little wonky. I had fat injections but they don't do very well. They tend to get reabsorbed." She posted a Twitter photo and story in July 2015, to show off her reconstruction and tattoo results, www .twitter.com/karenbrcamtl.

Preventive breast surgery remains "the biggest hot-button" issue among the women who frequent her BRCA Sisterhood website, she said.

"They want to know: Do I need to do this? How do I know if am making the right decision? The thing is, there is no right decision. It's a gamble. That's the biggest issue: How do we go from surveillance to actually making the decision to remove a healthy body part? My answer always is, there is no right answer. If I was the kind of person who could live with screenings every six months, and not be stressed, it would have been so much easier."

"Most women have a hard time and that's the biggest issue. How do you make that decision? You are petrified that you are going to get cancer. How do you get over that fear and do it? There's no answer."

"My advice is: If you are not sure about what you are going to do if you test positive, don't test for the mutation yet. Treat your body as if you are high risk. Go for your ultrasound or mammogram or MRI. People are so afraid about making these decisions. You don't get tested for the BRCA mutations because you want to remove your breasts. You don't have to do this. It's about due diligence and taking care of your health."

"What happens is women do surveillance for several years and then they realize the anxiety of waiting for those results is too difficult. That stress of, oh my God, this time they're going to find something. That's what changes the minds of a lot of people. I am getting emails from women who are 18, 19 and 20 and just finding out and they have no thoughts of surgery. They want children and families. That's where it becomes more difficult."

―――――⟪◉⟫―――――

A speech Kelly Rothe gave at Grand Valley University attracted a national filmmaker doing a documentary on hereditary breast cancer syndromes. She has a leading role in *Pink and Blue*, released in late 2015.

"I still can't fathom it," she said. "When he asked me to be the main feature in the film, I just walked around with a permanent smile on my face. It's crazy. It's a dream come true."

Going public "has been a sort of therapy, putting my story out there. I received thousands and thousands of well wishes. There were a few negative ones. But thousands of positive responses. When you have that many people praying for you and sending you good vibes, how could it do any harm?"

"I've learned a lot about myself," Rothe said. A month after her reconstruction in the fall of 2014, she resumed her studies in special education at Eastern Michigan University. "Eventually I want to go back to school and obtain my PhD to be an advocate for families and for students who have disabilities," she said. "That's my long-term plan."

Rothe underwent fertility preservation in July 2014, freezing seventeen eggs she someday may use in an in-vitro fertilization procedure. She already has decided that when she moves ahead to have children, she will undergo preimplantation genetic diagnosis, or PGD, that tests the DNA of the embryos and allows donors to implant only the eggs without gene abnormalities. "This gene stops with me," Rothe said.

In October 2014, Rothe had her fallopian tubes removed, leaving her ovaries after reading about recent studies "showing 60–100% of ovarian cancers start in the fallopian tubes," she said.

She plans to have other cancer prevention tests. "I'm going to go to the dermatologist to get my skin checked. I will get my regular colonoscopies. I have my physicals. I will do everything I can to protect myself against every type of cancer that I can."

She likes the results of her breast reconstruction, more than her original breasts. A friend who died of leukemia told her a phrase she likes to repeat about it: "It's worth it every day and twice on Sundays."

She added, "It's fantastic. Better than before. They are perkier. These are implants specifically made for women with mastectomies. They are gummy bears. Tear-drop shaped. They fit the contour of the natural breasts, compared to other implants that are round. They don't feel the same. I'm getting a lot of positive feedback from a couple of the groups I'm in online. We show pictures of our recovery. There are hundreds of comments."

"I won't be able to breastfeed my kids but I will be alive to have kids. And they are going to grow up with a mother."

Rothe counsels her younger sister about hereditary cancer. Her advice to her and others about a BRCA diagnosis: "It's not the end of the world.

You can go on and live life the way you normally would. You definitely can live with it." Referring to Angelina Jolie, she said: "To this day, I don't understand how she gets negative press for this. She chose to save her life. I know. I watched my mother suffer. And I essentially saw my younger brother and sister grow up without their mother. For me the chance to avoid that was worth it."

21

Family

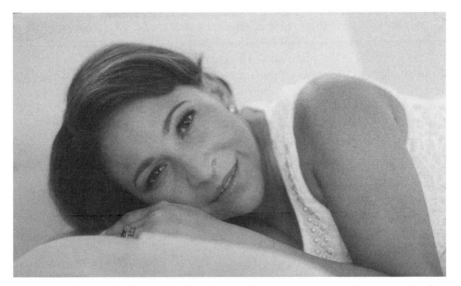

Ivy Hernandez was the first in her family to undergo genetic testing for cancer. She has spread word about the importance of testing to her extended family in Mexico.

Ivy Hernandez, a twenty-eight-year-old single mother at the time, inherited a big job when she found out she was a BRCA2 carrier.

As the first person in her family to be tested for a cancer mutation, Hernandez, now thirty-nine, of Newark, California, traveled to Mexico in 2014 to talk to her large family there. She has encouraged them to be tested to see if they, too, had the genetic mutation that significantly raises their risk of certain cancers, including breast, ovarian, pancreatic, and male breast tumors.

Within a year, thirteen relatives went in for genetic testing and counseling that she arranged for them to get by calling a large genetic testing company and asking for names of geneticists in Mexico.

Two cousins had preventive double mastectomies because they found they, too, carried the gene mutation. Others weren't interested, and many did not have health insurance and couldn't afford to pay for the tests or options they might pursue if they had the mutation.

"It's hard to give someone information when they can't do anything about it," Hernandez said. "What's the point of me telling them to get an MRI when they can't afford an MRI? Most of them don't have insurance. It's hard for them and for me, and I probably didn't talk about it with them as much as I'd like. I don't want to burden them with something they can't do much about."

These thorny family issues can be challenging and divisive. They also can leave some people feeling cursed while others blessed but almost guilty. At the same time, genetic findings can bring relief and enlightenment and can be a powerful bonding experience for many families.

The three oldest Rojas sisters of Anaheim and Santa Ana, California, have shared decisions about their prevention options ever since they were tested and found they carry the BRCA1 gene mutation that significantly raises their risk of breast and ovarian cancer. None has had cancer. A fourth sister, the youngest, does not carry the mutation.

Their mother, Alejandra Rojas, sixty-three, was diagnosed before she turned sixty with breast and ovarian cancer, three years apart. Her cancers led to her daughters' testing for the gene mutation and their eventual decisions to undergo preventive breast and ovarian cancer surgeries.

Socorro Rojas, thirty-two, a business analyst, had a total abdominal hysterectomy and bilateral salpingo-oophorectomy, removing her ovaries, uterus, and fallopian tubes in October 2014 and a nipple-sparing mastectomy with silicone implant reconstruction in November 2014. Her experience encouraged her older sister, Veronica, thirty-five, a Santa Ana schoolteacher, to meet with a genetic counselor and discuss her screening and prevention options to move ahead. She had the same preventive surgery as her sister, then had a nipple-sparing double mastectomy with silicone implant reconstruction on July 30, 2015 (chapter 3).

Erika Rojas Weinraub, twenty-nine, a Spanish translator, is pregnant and following cancer-screening guidelines for BRCA carriers.

The three older Rojas sisters attended the 2014 and 2015 annual conferences of Facing Our Risk Empowered, a large gathering of women with hereditary cancer syndromes that attracts some of the nation's top breast and gynecology specialists (www.facingourrisk.org). "I wanted to hear the new science and the new types of surgery," Veronica said.

Socorro and her husband attended the 2014 conference through a scholarship from FORCE. As a thank you, she started an Internet fundraiser that raised more than $1,650 for other scholarships, http://www .firstgiving.com/fundraiser/SocorroRojas/livelifeempowered. It carries

WATCHFUL WAITING

Many women with hereditary cancer syndromes choose what's known in medicine as watchful waiting or surveillance for a while or perhaps the rest of their lives.

The National Comprehensive Cancer Network, www.nccn.org, lists guidelines for cancer screening. But the decision is individualized, depending on a person's genetics and family history. Here are a few recommendations for women with a BRCA1 or 2 mutation:

- Clinical exam by a health care provider every six to twelve months and annual breast magnetic resonance imaging (MRI) beginning at age twenty-five.
- Annual mammography and breast MRI screening, commonly alternated every six months, beginning at age twenty-five or individualized based upon the earliest age of onset in the family.

a picture of the three sisters with their mother. "FORCE has empowered me to make life-changing medical decisions and I would love to give back," Socorro wrote. "With Angelina Jolie's recent revelation of being a BRCA carrier and having undergone a double mastectomy it is now more acceptable to talk about this very personal cause. My goal is to support FORCE in any way I can as they have been instrumental in my journey as a BRCA carrier. There needs to be more previvors hopefully like my sisters and I instead of more survivors like my mother or like two of her siblings who passed away from being carriers of this gene."

Forum Shah, a certified genetic counselor at St. Joseph Hospital in Orange, California, helps families understand their individual risk of cancer and the implications of a positive test result.

She remembers Veronica "seemed nervous and worried" when they met in 2014. "She thought perhaps I might insist she pick an option," Shah said. "I told her that's definitely not what I was there to do. I let her know that since she already had genetic testing, we could go straight into talking about her genetic test results. I said I was there to answer questions and to explain her results to her and what it means for her specifically. Once that was out of the way, I could tell Veronica just physically relaxed. I told Veronica, 'You've taken all the appropriate steps so far and have been doing all your screening.'"

=►◄(●)►◄=

GENETIC TESTING EXPLAINED

In an interview, Forum Shah, a genetics counselor at St. Joseph Hospital, Orange, California, discussed the increased interest in genetic testing, addressed common issues, and described the role of a genetics counselor.

Q: What impact did Angelina Jolie's 2013 statement have on interest in genetic testing?

A: I graduated the spring Angelina Jolie made her statement. More than anything, her statement brought awareness. BRCA testing has been clinically available for twenty years. Angelina Jolie made it more current news. So all these people who may have had genetic testing in the back of their minds starting thinking, maybe I should be doing this right now. Increased awareness has led to a significant growth in the number of patients we are seeing and in the number of counselors needed. A lot of centers thought one genetic counselor was enough, or even a part-time genetics counselor. Now they are hiring three to four at some centers because we're seeing the increase in awareness.

Q: Who is coming in to be tested?

A: The youngest patient that I've seen was sixteen years old; the oldest was eighty-five. The patient demographic depends on each individual's story and their reasons for coming in for a genetic consultation. You have women recently diagnosed with breast cancer, from thirty to seventy. You have women who were diagnosed with breast cancer years ago, when they were in their thirties and now they are in their sixties and seventies. Their daughter brought up this issue with them and they are worried. We always think the most informative person to test is the person affected at a young age with cancer.

Q: How early can testing begin?

A: Usually genetic testing is available at eighteen years of age. However, many individuals choose to wait until twenty-five years of age as screening is generally not started before twenty-five years. There are some genetic syndromes we will test for earlier at younger ages because the screening for those syndromes is recommended to start at an earlier age.

Q: What is the cost of testing, and has it become more affordable?

A: Insurance is more likely to cover genetic testing now compared to several years ago. We have insurance criteria to follow. The criteria are considered to be in most cases what we call fair and valid. They are based on research that shows that women with breast cancer forty-five years of age and younger are at a higher risk to have a hereditary predisposition. Research has also shown that women sixty years of age and younger with triple-negative breast cancer have a higher risk to carry a hereditary predisposition. Insurance plans have different criteria. Depending on the plan's criteria, a patient may have an obstacle. Medicare, for example, does not cover testing in unaffected individuals. When a younger woman tests positive for a genetic mutation we want to know if she inherited her mutation from her mother or her father so the family members can be informed. If her parents have Medicare and are unaffected, it becomes harder to test them as they would have to pay for the test themselves.

Q: So most people have insurance to cover this?

A: Most people do. If they don't, we have great resources. Each laboratory has its own financial resources that they perhaps can offer. Myriad used to be the only company to test for BRCA1 and 2. Since its patent was dissolved by a Supreme Court ruling, the price of genetic testing has gone down significantly. It was about $4,400.

Q: And now?

A: Depending on which laboratory you go to, and which panel of tests, it can be $2,000 or less.

Q: And subsequent family members are charged less?

A: Yes, once someone has tested positive for a mutation, then we test others in the family for that mutation. We call this single-site testing, which is less expensive, about $300 to $400. If someone wants to pay out of pocket because of insurance or other reasons, many labs have discounts on testing for less.

Q: Do some companies charge less?

A: Beyond BRCA1 and 2 testing, we can order any panel for $1,500 or less in out-of-pocket costs.

Q: What does a variant of uncertain significance (VUS) result mean?

A: Besides a positive or negative result, the laboratory can also detect what is known as a variant of uncertain significance. This happens maybe 10 percent of the time in panel testing. Historically, about 90 percent of VUS results in BRCA carriers were reclassified as benign.

Q: Are there other genes associated with breast cancer?

A: Although the BRCA1 and 2 genes are the most common causes of hereditary breast cancer, they are not the only known causes of hereditary breast cancer. Other high-risk genetic syndromes are rare but they exist. Many genes, like PALB2, are associated with a moderately higher risk of breast cancer. We discuss panel testing with all women during a genetic consultation. We emphasize panel testing as a personal choice if patients want to do testing for moderate-risk genes. Standard management guidelines for these moderate-risk genes have not been developed yet. We encourage everyone, including our BRCA patients, to be part of a study because that's the only way we are going to gather more information. Some of these studies are looking at particular mutations. Right now, we give ranges. Certain mutations may have more or less of a penetrance and therefore the increased risk to cancer varies. That's why we encourage women to go into research, whenever they are ready. That's how we are able to get these risks to begin with.

Q: What is BART (BRACAnalysis® Rearrangement Test)?

A: BART is a test that adds to the extra accuracy of BRCA1 and 2 sequencing tests, making the combination of the two tests 97 percent accurate. A sequencing test reads the letters of a person's genetic code to see if there are any typos or errors; was anything misspelled? What BART testing does is to indicate if there are portions of the gene missing or extra. This is called duplication/deletion testing because it looks for missing or duplicated areas within a gene. We know a harmful error can cause the gene to no longer function, and that's what we call a positive result—the patient has inherited a hereditary predisposition to cancer.

Q: Do many people get the BART test?

A: Now, BART is a standard of care when testing for the BRCA1 and BRCA2 genes is ordered. Anyone who has had a genetic counseling consultation since 2013 to do BRCA testing will have sequencing and deletion/duplication testing. Between 2006 and 2012, some patients were tested; some were not. So we are always encouraging patients to contact us if it's been two to three years since they were last seen to determine if they qualify for additional testing.

Q: What does BART cost?

A: It's about $700.

Q: If someone in your family has had BART testing, do you still need it?

A: It would depend. It's a tricky question. If someone in your family already had BART testing and they were affected with a young cancer, and you were unaffected, then no, you don't need it. If you are affected with cancer and someone else in the family has had BART testing, and you are the youngest person affected with cancer in the family, then yes, we'd want you to do the test.

We don't test everyone we see. We are genetic counselors. We educate people about genetics. We do a risk assessment. We look at their family history. We determine if testing is necessary. We interpret test results for them. There are women who walk out of my office who don't get testing done. We talk and they decide, "I don't need this testing. I can save the money." But they can walk out reassured. They can say, "I'm not ignoring this family history. I know it exists. It's definitely concerning. Here's what we're going to do about it." We have risk models to help calculate what the chance of a person developing cancer is given the personal and family history.

Q: Is depression common when learning you are BRCA positive, even if you are educated and motivated to learn your results?

A: It depends. The beneficial aspect about counseling prior to testing is that you can talk about it with your patients and prepare them before they choose to pursue testing. Have you thought about what it is like to be positive? Have you thought about what it is like to be negative? You allow the patients to start thinking about positive test results. I have a lot of people who come in and say, "I already know I am positive. I am going to think that so that if I test negative, I will be getting good news and if I'm positive, I'm preparing for that." It works both ways. I can tell someone they are negative and they start crying. "I wasn't expecting it." I think my negative patients cry more often than my positive patients because they are so stunned and surprised. It's so unexpected for them.

Q: Do you give results over the phone?

A: It depends on the patient and how comfortable the patients feel about receiving the news over the phone. If the results are positive, we strongly advise the patients return for a follow-up appointment within a few days of receiving the news. This gives them a day or two to adjust to the results. It's like hearing you have cancer. You hear the word and nothing else. It's the same sometimes when you hear you are positive. You don't necessarily hear what goes with it. So sometimes it's nice to give the news over the phone and they have a day or two to adjust. When they come in, they are armed with questions and knowledge.

Q: If a woman has breast cancer, she may use genetic results to decide whether to have a contralateral prophylactic mastectomy. How do you counsel women about that, given the fact that the surgery doesn't help a woman live longer?

A: It depends on how a woman feels when she comes in. I tell her, you are positive for a BRCA mutation and your risk of developing a second primary breast cancer is 40 to 60 percent. I say it's up to you whether you want to keep the second breast. I ask, "If you are positive for a BRCA mutation, do you go in for your mammograms and clinical breast exams?"

If the person is negative, we say it's one-half of a percent every year until age eighty. At that point I ask, "Are you someone who is vigilant about screening? Your physician is going to watch you like a hawk for the first five to ten years anyway. After that, are you going to continue to be vigilant?"

You have other patients who say, "I don't want to do all this screening. I'm going to stress every single day of my life over the fact that I still have my other breast." Sometimes, you have to weigh the emotional distress with the surgery complications and recovery. If emotionally, every day of their life they are thinking about whether they are going to develop breast cancer in the other breast, I don't know how beneficial it is to keep the other breast.

I always tell women that I cannot tell them about recurrence risks from their first cancer. That's something to discuss with their oncologist. I am talking to them about a completely new risk. I always emphasize with anyone who walks into this door that even if you remove both of your breasts, your risk of developing breast cancer is not going to be zero. Nothing takes it down to 0 percent. Breast tissue could still exist in the chest wall.

Q: Of women who are positive, do more choose surveillance than treatment?

A: It's a very unique personal choice. It's hard to say. It may be age dependent and may depend on whether they have cancer or not. When someone is unaffected and young, they tend to make statements like, "I want to breastfeed. I want to keep my breasts for a while. I'm going to do screening." What I tell all my unaffected patients is that studies show if a woman vigilantly does her screening—mammograms and MRIs every year; clinical breast exams every six months—versus a woman who does a bilateral mastectomy, what we found is their survival is the same.

I say, "This is information for when or if you are ready." At the end of the session, I always ask if a patient feels comfortable doing testing as it may change their life. I've had some who have walked out saying, "Thank you for all the knowledge. I'm not ready right now. I don't think I want this test right now but I will do my screening." That's all I want. I want them to do their screening.

Q: How much does a BRCA1 or 2 mutation raise a person's risk of breast and ovarian cancer?

A: It raises the risk of breast cancer by up to 85 percent and of ovarian by up to 45 percent. Ovarian cancer risk depends on which gene mutation you are carrying. BRCA1 raises ovarian cancer risk by up to 45 percent; a BRCA2 mutation raises the risk to up to 20 percent. For breast cancer, we don't differentiate between the two. We say the risk of developing a primary breast cancer is between 56 to 85 percent. For a second primary breast cancer, it's 40 to 60 percent.

Q: If a woman is BRCA1 or 2 positive, when do you recommend she remove her ovaries? And when should screening begin when someone else in your family has cancer at a young age?

A: We generally recommend you remove your ovaries by age forty. If you have had your children, you can remove them earlier if you want. After you hit forty years of age, your risk starts getting higher.

We suggest screening should begin ten years before the youngest cancer in the family. For example, if someone had breast cancer at thirty-five years of age, we recommend their family members start breast screening at twenty-five years of age. If someone has ovarian cancer at thirty-five years of age, we will be a little more concerned as currently, but there is no data to support ovarian cancer screening.

Q: How do genetic counselors assist other family members about test results?

A: Once someone is positive, I focus on what these results mean for my patient. Oftentimes, we use charts, graphs, or pictures to aid in the explanations. Such as, "Here is the risk to the general population. Here is the risk group in which you are falling. You are falling into this high-risk group." We talk to our patients about what the numbers mean.

We give them a chart, and we give them a list of the National Comprehensive Cancer Network guidelines, which goes over how we want to screen them. Some of it is split by age, some by gender. Then we go on to the family. Even if you come in for yourself, at the end of the day testing has implications for other family members. We always take a family history when a patient comes in. It includes parents, siblings, aunts, uncles, grandparents, cousins. We have letters we give people they can take to family members to discuss the tests. Anyone can come in and talk to us.

Shah explains the implications of testing, including several important issues facing younger women. "Removing your ovaries before age 35 cuts your risk of breast cancer in half," Shah said. "But you have to talk about the fact that it's going to put you into early menopause. Are you ready for that? When you surgically take out the ovaries, it brings instant menopause. There is no slow progression into menopause. When you are in your twenties and thirties, your sexual life is very active. To be put into menopause instantly brings sexual changes as well. There can be dryness. You may not feel those sexual needs as easily and quickly as you did prior to the surgery. It's not a topic that is talked about as often. Patients are shy to talk about it. There may be self-image issues. Yes, women will get new, perky breasts but those breasts aren't their own breasts. Women may have difficulty adjusting to this change. Some have issues because of that. Some women are scared and don't know whether to take hormone replacement therapy. I go into some of the pros and cons of things that go into these decisions. Part of our job is to help women come to terms with these risks. We can't answer all of the medical questions, at which time we encourage the patients to talk to their other care providers, including their surgeons. Shah tells patients, 'Part of this process is asking for help and saying, I can't do this alone. I need to ask the experts.'"

Shah also gave the Rojas family a letter they translated into Spanish for their relatives. Alejandra Rojas took the letter on a trip in July 2015 to see relatives in Oaxaca, Mexico. She planned another trip in October and will bring more letters for her extended family. "We are the first ones in our family to know we are positive," Erika said. "It's hard to explain."

"In our family the younger ones who have more knowledge and who've been to college, they understand. Others who are less educated, they don't want it. Some say, 'what's the point, we're going to die.' That's why I have taken it upon myself to contact everyone and make them aware. It's their choice whether they want to get tested."

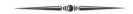

Conveying genetic news to family members who live abroad brings other issues. Some relatives might not have health insurance or can't afford to pay for tests or surgery options, and that brings a twinge of remorse.

"I was born here," said Hernandez. "Most of my family lives in Mexico. The access to health care I have is not there for them like I have. I have been very lucky. I was the first one to get tested. I talked about it a lot with my family. I think in the last two years everything started changing a little bit. I was actually able to find a place in Mexico to help. I sent one of my family members over there who got breast cancer. Thank goodness, this doctor decided to use my whole family as a study."

"My family is a very old generation. It's mostly my cousins getting tested, and their kids. I don't know what they'll do with the information. Two of my cousins decided to go the surgery route who are over 50. It's an easier thing then. I'm more worried about my other nephews and nieces. They don't have the access to the health care I do. They might test positive, but what do we do then? Is testing a good thing then?"

Hernandez recalled at least ten relatives who died of one sort of cancer or another. "We knew something was wrong in the family. We traced it to my mom's dad, who came from Spain. We don't know much about him. We don't know much about his heritage. I traced my mutation back to Finland."

Because she wanted another child, Hernandez chose to monitor her cancer risk for seven years with mammograms, MRIs, and the ovarian cancer CA-125 blood test. "I have a great team of doctors. Everyone was cheerful with me and extra cautious. They'd remind me, it's time for this, it's time for that. Maybe I was their guinea pig. I didn't mind the MRIs, the ultrasounds and the mammograms. I knew it was for the best for me."

Her Catholic religion also was an issue in her choice to not have surgery initially. "Religion is a big deal. You think, who am I to be fixing something? You're kind of playing God in a way. It didn't stop me, but it did pop into my head. Should I leave it up to Him to help me through it? And I think that could be the same with any religion out there."

Hernandez had her second child in 2012, and shortly afterward, she was diagnosed with ductal carcinoma in situ, an early stage tumor. She had a bilateral nipple-sparing mastectomy with silicone implant reconstruction on July 7, 2013.

"Everything worked out," she said. "I'm very small chested. That's why I was able to do nipple sparing. It was very early on so I had no chemo or radiation. It went smoothly. I was very lucky. The only small complication I had was a little bit of necrosis on my nipples. I was warned ahead of time. I didn't lose them. They look fine. I do like them." She wears more halter than V-neck shirts to hide the dent, as she calls it, or distortion that occurs in her implants when she lifts or bends her arms.

Still, she said of her old breasts, "I miss them dearly, very, very much. More than anything it's the sensitivity side that I miss the most. Lookwise, I'm not very concerned. It's more an issue with the loss of sensitivity."

She also had her fallopian tubes removed, along with one ovary, hoping to avoid being pushed into menopause when both ovaries are taken. "I was thirty-seven at mastectomy; I had reconstruction at thirty-nine; I am not ready for any other surgery. I'm a single mom with a busy work life. I can't deal with losing my estrogen to keep my sanity. I want to be happy." She has the CA-125 test every six months to watch for cancer. "Sixty percent of ovarian cancers start in the tubes and I don't need my tubes any more," she said. "So they removed my tubes but I kept one ovary."

Hernandez is glad to know she has the mutation. She doesn't see it as a burden. "I guess it doesn't scare me," she said. "For me, it's like hey, I know what I have. At least I know about it. I knew it was coming. Still, you say, oh my gosh. Fear is a huge thing that strikes first. Choosing the surveillance route allowed me to get a lot of my fears and demons out. It's my personal opinion; nowadays a lot of people are getting tested. Then if they get positive results, they go for surgery when they might not be emotionally ready," she said.

"I think the best thing is to be at ease and accepting of the diagnosis before you go ahead. The surgeries are so overwhelming. And if there are complications you can break down. I never had surgery in my life. I was very small-chested. I had always wanted big boobs. I've never thought about doing it. Both my kids were natural births. I never even had anesthesia. It's overwhelming. It is a huge surgery. You come out feeling there's an elephant on your chest. The pressure is horrible. I was very lucky it all went right. I can't imagine someone who just tested positive two months ago and goes into surgery without processing it correctly and then having complications."

Hernandez plans to let her daughter decide about testing by herself. "I'll leave it up to her. She is very knowledgeable about it. She knows I'm positive. She saw me go through the surgery. I've talked to her but I don't go into much detail. She can't get tested until she is eighteen anyway. If they offer her the test at eighteen, I don't know if she will. Knowing her, she may wait till her early twenties. Hopefully in the coming years there will be more options for her."

"My son is three and hopefully by the time he is eighteen things will have changed and there will be better options. I really don't want to worry about him."

She hopes the discussion about genetics moves beyond surgery issues to better understanding how to live with a higher risk of cancer.

"The Angelina effect created awareness, but I think everyone takes it as a push towards surgery and that's it. In fact, unfortunately, surgery doesn't take all the risk away. I still have the mutation. It is something I live with. There should be more talk about how to live with it. I think that's something that's missing. I heard someone say, 'I am going to have surgery. I just want to get it over.' But you still have to live with it."

"I don't let it define me. I'm not defective. I have a bad gene I need to deal with, but we all do. At least I know about it."

22

Pregnancy

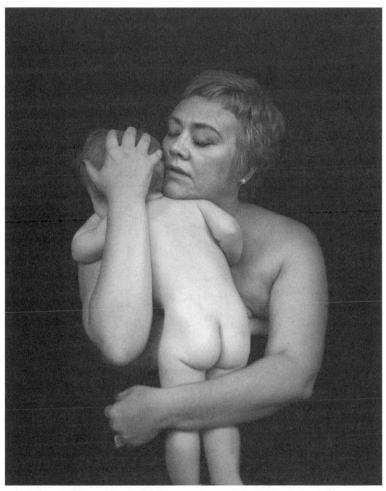

Sara Erzen found a lump in her breast while pregnant with her third child, but she had to convince her doctor to order tests that confirmed it was cancer.

Sara Erzen regularly asked her doctors during the first five months of her pregnancy about the lump in her left breast.

When it persisted and got painful and she kept asking about it, her doctor ordered tests that eventually led to her diagnosis with an aggressive stage 3 tumor.

She needed chemotherapy, surgery, and radiation, all sandwiched around the birth of her daughter, Adeline Faith, in March 2014. During the same operation, she had her ovaries removed to ensure cancer didn't spread. Then she switched medical teams from Lansing to Detroit.

In all, Erzen, a one-time emergency medical technician, clocked 176.5 hours and 10,271 miles traveling to metro Detroit from her home in Holt, Michigan, ninety miles away, for her cancer treatments and breast cancer surgery and reconstruction.

She counted each health care interaction: "65 appointments; 8 rounds of chemo; 3 ER visits; 31 different medications; 4 hospitalizations; 5 surgeries; 104 tests; and 30 radiation treatments."

Worth it? Without question, said Erzen, thirty-seven, a full-time homemaker with two other daughters from a previous marriage. "I'm hoping to never have a year like the one we just went through again. But I'm well and living life."

As little as two decades ago, doctors did not prescribe cancer treatments during pregnancy, and many counseled women to end a pregnancy if they had cancer, according to research published by the Cancer and Pregnancy Registry at the Cooper Medical School, Camden, New Jersey.[1]

Research from the registry and elsewhere has helped doctors gain confidence that they can give chemotherapy drugs to pregnant women that won't harm their babies.

Chemotherapy given during pregnancy does not adversely affect a child's cognitive skills, academic achievement, or behavioral competence compared to children not exposed to chemotherapy, according to the New Jersey registry, started in 1997 to track maternal and fetal outcomes after a cancer diagnosis in pregnancy.

"There's a comfort level that it's safe to give chemo to women as more and more healthy babies are born," though medicine still lacks big studies about the effect of chemotherapy during pregnancy on both the woman and fetus, explained Dr. Haythem Ali, Erzen's medical oncologist in the Henry Ford Health System, Detroit.

As women delay having children, more breast cancer is likely to be diagnosed during pregnancy, the National Cancer Institute says.

Currently, breast cancer occurs in 1 of every 3,000 pregnancies. It is the most common of all tumors diagnosed during pregnancy, followed by hematological cancers such as leukemia, according to the NCI.[2]

Other women are diagnosed with breast cancer shortly after giving birth, including while lactating, or in subsequent months when childbirth may trigger higher estrogen production and possibly fuel a tumor.

Many women are diagnosed late, on average five to fifteen months from the onset of symptoms, because "the natural tenderness and engorgement of the breasts of pregnant and lactating women may hinder detection," the NCI said. The agency says:

- Pregnant women should perform breast self-exams and undergo a clinician exam by a doctor during pregnancy.
- Mammography and biopsies are safe to be performed in pregnancy.
- Overall survival of pregnant women with breast cancer may be worse than in nonpregnant women, but that "may be primarily the result of delayed diagnosis."
- Termination of pregnancy "has not been shown to have any beneficial effect on breast cancer outcome and is not considered as a therapeutic option."

While treatment options for women diagnosed with cancer during pregnancy have grown, resources and consumer sources of information are sparse. One nonprofit, Hope for Two: The Pregnant with Cancer Network, http://www.hopefortwo.org/, shares stories of pregnant women with different types of cancer diagnosed in pregnancy and connects women with a shared diagnosis.

Erzen's story explains some of the most common issues women face during pregnancy: the difficulties of detecting cancer during pregnancy; how cancer affects the timing of breast surgery and reconstruction; and the issues women may face if they have reconstruction.

⸻⸻◉⸻⸻

At thirty-seven, Erzen was delighted to be pregnant. She and her new husband, James, a firefighter and paramedic, wanted another child.

Just before the pregnancy was confirmed, she noticed a hard spot in her left breast. She said she told her obstetrician about it at each of her monthly prenatal appointments, for the first five months of her pregnancy. Each time, she said, doctor and nurses reassured her with phrases like, "'Well you are young. You have dense breast tissue. You may end up lactating more' where she found the lump," she said.

Finally, even though she was told "there's nothing to worry about," her doctor ordered an ultrasound test. A letter arrived telling her, in capital letters, she had "NO ABNORMALITIES." But it didn't ease her fears because "by then I started waking up in the middle of the night in pain. My husband would get up to make me hot compresses" to put on her chest for relief, she said. On her next prenatal appointment, she asked a nurse to take another look.

"I took my bra off. I said, 'I want you to feel this. It just doesn't seem right.' She felt it and said, if you want, we'll refer you to a breast surgeon." She got a referral to see the specialist, but she had to wait two weeks to get in to see him.

Erzen was five months pregnant when she saw the surgeon in November. By then, she found two more lumps in her breast and axilla, she said. He asked her to remove her shirt and began feeling the more prominent lump. She remembered him asking her, "How long have you had this?" she said. She told him how she had tried throughout her pregnancy to point out the lump.

"He excused himself from the room and came in with another doctor. He told the second physician, 'I want you to feel this.' Then he said, 'You are going for a biopsy right now. I will call the office and let them know you are coming.'"

Before leaving, she asked the surgeon, "'I want you to tell me what you are seeing right now.' He said, 'Well I can tell you there are good options for chemotherapy during pregnancy.' That's how we knew. We knew when we went for the biopsy that I had cancer."

The biopsy confirmed a stage 3 tumor that had spread to several sentinel lymph nodes. She needed chemotherapy before surgery to shrink the tumors, then surgery and radiation.

She called her parents, who had just left Michigan to spend the winter in Florida. "Within 48 hours, they packed up their RV and they were back in Michigan."

In shock, without thinking, Erzen posted a notice on Facebook about her diagnosis. "I got a call from the counselor at school," Erzen said. A friend of her oldest daughter, Katey, ten at the time, had heard from her mother that Erzen had cancer.

"It was a horrible way to find out," Katey said. "I started talking to this girl. Her mom is on Facebook with my mom. She comes up, pats me on the back and says, 'oh yah, your mom has breast cancer.'"

Erzen and her daughter had a long talk when they got home. Katey said, "I had been seeing her crying a lot. I knew something wasn't right."

Erzen's memory of the traumatic day is a little blurry. "I think I said something like, 'it is what it is. I'm going to be ok. I'm going to lose my hair. I'm probably going to lose my breasts. I'm going to be sick but I have to do this. We've got this baby coming. I'm pretty sure I said, we have to all pull together as a family.'"

Angry and a little shocked, Erzen switched doctors. An aunt who is a home health care provider recommended the Henry Ford Health System in Detroit. Within a few days the hospital's tumor board reviewed her case and recommended adjuvant chemotherapy before surgery, a mastectomy, and radiation. Erzen met with a multidisciplinary medical team that explained her treatment plan that included a breast surgeon, a medical oncologist, a maternal-fetal medicine specialist, and a radiation oncologist.

When breast cancer is diagnosed in a pregnant woman, "your primary concern is the mother," Ali said. "She needs to have the best possible treatment to ensure her survival. You want to make sure all options are open to the mother. But you also want to make sure you don't harm this new life as much as you can, to minimize the risk to the baby as well. So there's this delicate balance to do the best for the mother as best as you can and have a healthy baby delivered."

Chemotherapy is safe when delivered after the first trimester, he said. Still, doctors use older chemotherapy drugs with known side effects during pregnancy and save newer medicine for afterward, he said. "We split the drugs into ones we feel comfortable with and ones we don't," Ali said. "Drugs like Adriamycin that we've given since the seventies and that we know, we will use in pregnancy while newer drugs such as taxanes that we don't really understand their effects, we try to wait to use those drugs until after the baby is delivered. You don't want to risk having a malformed organ. You have to make sure you are balancing the mother's health with the safety of the child."

Medicine has never been able to study cancer drugs given during pregnancy because it would be unethical to create studies giving medicines to one group of pregnant women and not another, Ali said. "There is an ethical issue here that you can't overcome," he said. "So the information is from women, reporting back their experiences. It's sort of like climbing Mt. Everest. You have to find your way. There was hardly any information ten to fifteen years ago. Even now, the information is largely based on experience, not what we like to see in medicine, which is clinical trials."

Erzen completed a second round of chemotherapy and soon was ready for a unilateral mastectomy with silicone implant reconstruction on June 25, 2014. In the same surgery, doctors removed twenty-one lymph nodes, and they placed a tissue expander in her chest as the first step in implant reconstruction.

Within two weeks, Erzen made the first of several trips to the emergency department for an infection in her breast from the expanders. She had to be hospitalized then readmitted when the infection persisted. When it finally resolved, Erzen started thirty rounds of daily radiation, finishing December 12, 2014.

Throughout it all, she gained strength and support from family, church, friends, and online support groups. She grew to appreciate that she was alive and happy. She wants to keep it that way and doesn't want to risk any problems returning for reconstruction.

"I'm not pursuing reconstruction at this time," Erzen said in July 2015. "It's not a big deal. I've embraced the change in my body and I am focused on being a role model for my three daughters. If nothing else, I hope this experience shows them that they can love the skin they're in, no matter the circumstance."

Her oldest daughter, Katey, said her mother's strength throughout the entire last year motivates the entire family. "Now I know she's going to be OK," Katey said. "Over time, I've learned more about it so it's not as scary. And I know she's very strong. She's really strong because she never said, 'oh my gosh, I have cancer. I'm going to die.' She said, 'I can battle this. I'm not going to let this get in my way.'"

23

Wrapping It Up

Breast cancer surgery or reconstruction can be daunting and confusing. Surgery decisions may feel urgent, or you may feel pressured to make choices quickly. It may seem hard making up your mind, given how you feel and all the issues to consider. Later, how do you go about addressing other remaining issues, and how do you get your life back to something like it was?

Here are the best suggestions we have collected from women, doctors, and other resources to help you make good, informed choices.

THE DIAGNOSIS

Once you learn you have breast cancer or carry a mutation that greatly raises your risk of getting it, many women feel pressured to move quickly. They want to move on, as many say. In fact, most wait to have reconstruction. That gives you time to sort out some of the confusion. If you search the Internet for answers, try not to get overwhelmed by all the information.

ASSEMBLING YOUR PERSONAL AND MEDICAL TEAMS

Ask your doctor, family, and friends for names of breast surgeons and, if desired, plastic surgeons. Visit doctor or hospital websites. The best teams have extensive information online about their practices, the surgery options they perform, and pictures of patients with breast reconstruction.

Find someone who is a good listener to bring with you to your first appointment with your surgeon or medical team. If no one is available, bring a small tape recorder to the appointment and ask to use it. Bring any questions you have with you. Don't be afraid to ask to have information repeated or explained. You also need to ask the doctor, hospital, or your insurance plan what out-of-pocket costs you face. If your health plan doesn't cover all costs and you have a limited income, you may be eligible for help from a few nonprofit organizations, such as The Pink Fund and My Hope Chest, listed below with other resources.

Take time, too, to see how the doctor reacts to your questions. Is she comfortable with you asking for information? Does she explain issues clearly? Ask to see pictures of a doctor's patients or bring a picture of your breasts or ones you like and ask if the doctor can give you new breasts like your old ones or others you like. Request names of patients you can call and visit, or find breast cancer survivors in your area who will talk to you and even may show you their breasts. If you don't like how the doctor responds, find another one, preferably at another hospital where practice patterns and options may be different.

Ask if you are eligible for surgery advances, such as direct-to-implant, one-step reconstruction, or a nipple-sparing mastectomy. What kind of incisions does the doctor typically use, and what kind of scars will you be left with? If you are having reconstruction, find out if the plastic surgeon mostly performs reconstruction with implants, as most do. Find out if you are at higher risk of surgery complications, such as lymphedema, heart problems caused by radiation to breast tumors in the left breast over the heart, and other issues. If you are at risk, what precautions do you and the doctor need to follow? Do you need a test to find out whether you have a higher risk for problems?

YOUR HOMEWORK

It is important to be in the best physical shape possible before surgery. Stop smoking, if you do, because it increases the risk of complications. You may even have to pass a nicotine test at some hospitals before surgery is scheduled. Lose weight if possible because obesity is associated with a higher rate of surgery problems. Find a caregiver or team you can rely on to get you to appointments, help with household tasks, or mind your pets. Some women create Internet pages that allow family and friends to get updates about you and to sign up for bringing you meals or helping with other tasks. Pack items you need to take to the hospital, such as a robe, a comfortable surgery bra or abdominal binder if you have breast reconstruction with abdominal tissue, and a pillow to place on your chest or tummy under a seat belt for your ride home. This also is the time to take care of items you may not be able to tend to for a while. Get your hair cut or colored, get a pedicure, and shave or wax your legs or underarms, as you may not be able to do those activities for a few weeks. Pet owners also may want to consider arrangements, perhaps elsewhere if possible, for their animals, because they may jump on your chest or expose you to bacteria while you are recovering in the first few weeks.

POSTSURGERY

Your first few weeks after surgery may be challenging. Many women feel they or their doctors underestimate or underplay recovery issues. Some doctors and women suggest scheduling more recovery time from work or normal activities than you think you may need.

At home, follow instructions carefully about the surgery drains you may have. Keep track of the fluid drainage and avoid getting the drains wet. Some doctors say no showering until the drains are removed; others allow showering with precautions, such as showering backward for a few weeks. Some doctors and women recommend purchasing a new or used shower chair to help caregivers help you shower. Wear the postsurgery bra you purchased or the hospital provided for you until your drains are removed. Rest and sleep on your back, propped up to be comfortable. If you are in severe pain, have lots of swelling, or running a high temperature, call your doctor's office for help.

It will take weeks, even months, to get back to normal activities or feel comfortable with your new body. You may feel weird sensations, such as a pulling sensation, or be unable to lift your arm, even to take a half-gallon container of milk out of the refrigerator in the week or two after surgery. Your skin may swell a little or look like an orange peel with larger pores, a common problem caused by swelling. Your nipple, if you have one, may develop a scab, change color or shape. Your breasts also may feel tight or too high up on your chest, which should resolve over the next few months. Gentle breast massages may help, beginning about two weeks after surgery, to increase blood flow and reduce swelling. Dab lotion on your fingers once or twice a day and gently massage your breasts. In the meantime, don't use heat pads or ice packs as both can damage the skin. With time, sometimes weeks or even months, swelling should resolve. Back pain also is common because you can't sleep on your chest or side, in ways your body is not accustomed. Begin walking, even around the house for a few minutes.

Two weeks after surgery, most women can begin light exercises to increase their range of motion in their arms once or twice a day. These exercises are simple movements, such as walking your hands up a wall as if you were washing it. Other exercises also can begin, but don't overdo it. Walking, running, and using exercise machines that don't require much arm movement should be fine, in moderation. Exercises such as push-ups, weightlifting, swimming, and yoga aren't typically advised for a few months. If you still are having problems, you may need physical therapy, which your doctor has to prescribe. Some doctors recommend avoiding hot tubs for six months because of exposure to bacteria.

MENTAL HEALTH

Consider joining a support group. Many hospitals have them for breast cancer patients or can refer you to one in your area. Be honest with yourself if you are feeling really down. Some studies suggest that depression, even thoughts of suicide, is more common in women after breast cancer surgery than many think. Talk to your doctor immediately if you feel that way and ask for help. If you have a partner and develop problems, consider counseling as well. If you are sexually active, avoid placing too much weight on incisions. If you are part of online support groups, try not to get overwhelmed with what might seem like a barrage of sometimes conflicting information and opinions.

BEST OVERALL RESOURCES

American Society of Plastic Surgeons, Breast Reconstruction Planner, http://static1.squarespace.com/static/55a930ffe4b0e82a77493f6f/t/55c e1cd8e4b06614877a84ad/1439571160239/breast-reconstruction-recovery -guide-planner.pdf
   Cancer Prevention and Treatment Fund, http://www.stopcancerfund .org/prevention/breast-cancer/
   Facing Our Risk of Cancer Empowered, FORCE, www.facingourrisk .org
   National Cancer Institute, www.cancer.gov
   Young Survival Coalition, www.youngsurvival.org

BEST RESOURCES, OTHER ISSUES

Breast implants: www.fda.gov
   Financial help: The Pink Fund, www.pinkfund; My Hope Chest, www .myhopechest.org
   Nutrition: Diana Dyer, registered dietitian and breast cancer survivor, http://www.dianadyer.com; Annie Appleseed Project, http://www .annieappleseedproject.org

Notes

CHAPTER 1: MODERN BREAST SURGERY AND RECONSTRUCTION

1. Angelina Jolie, "My Medical Choice," *New York Times*, May 14, 2013, http://www.nytimes.com/2013/05/14/opinion/my-medical-choice.html?_r=0.

2. Department of Labor, "Your Rights After a Mastectomy," http://www.dol.gov/ebsa/publications/whcra.html.

3. Meeghan Lautner et al., "Disparities in the Use of Breast-Conserving Therapy Among Patients with Early-Stage Breast Cancer," *JAMA Surgery* 150, no. 8 (2015), http:/archsurg.jamanetwork.com/article.aspx?articleid=2322835.

4. American Society of Plastic Surgeons, 2014 Plastic Surgery Statistics, http://www.plasticsurgery.org/news/plastic-surgery-statistics/2014-statistics.html.

5. Monica Morrow et al., "Access to Breast Reconstruction After Mastectomy and Patient Perspectives on Reconstruction Decision Making," *JAMA Surgery* 149, no. 10 (2014): 1015–21.

6. Lautner et al., "Disparities in the Use of Breast-Conserving Therapy."

7. National Institutes of Health, "Treatment of Early-Stage Breast Cancer," Consensus Development Conference Statement, June 18–21, 1990, https://consensus.nih.gov/1990/1990earlystagebreastcancer081html.htm.

8. SSSO-ASTRO Consensus Guideline, "Margins for Breast-Conserving Surgery with Whole Breast Irradiation in Stage I and II Invasive Breast Cancer," http://www.surgonc.org/docs/default-source/pdf/sso-astro_consensus_guideline_on_margins_for_breast_conserving_surgery_final.pdf?sfvrsn=2.

9. Judith Medeiros Fitzgerald, *A Teacher's Journey . . . What Breast Cancer Taught Me* (CreateSpace Independent Publishing, 2012), https://www.createspace.com/3751875.

10. Ford Motor Company, Warriors in Pink, http://warriorsinpink.ford.com/models-of-courage/model/view/id/12#sthash.UjqliRFu.dpuf.

CHAPTER 2: MAKING THE DECISION

1. U.S. Food and Drug Administration, "Regulatory History of Breast Implants in the U.S.," http://www.fda.gov/MedicalDevices/ProductsandMedicalProcedures/ImplantsandProsthetics/BreastImplants/ucm064461.htm.

2. Meeghan Lautner et al., "Disparities in the Use of Breast-Conserving Therapy Among Patients with Early-Stage Breast Cancer," *JAMA Surgery*, July 17, 2005. http://archsurg.jamanetwork.com/article.aspx?articleid=2322835.

3. National Institutes of Health, "Treatment of Early-Stage Breast Cancer," Consensus Development Conference Statement, June 18–21, 1990, https://consensus.nih.gov/1990/1990earlystagebreastcancer081html.htm.

4. National Comprehensive Cancer Network, http://www.nccn.org/patients/guidelines/stage_i_ii_breast/index.html.

5. Steven A. Narod et al., "Breast Cancer Mortality After a Diagnosis of Ductal Carcinoma in Situ," *JAMA Oncology* 1, no. 17 (October 2015). doi:10.1001/jamaoncol.2015.2510.

6. Dunya Atisha et al., "Prospective Analysis of Long-Term Psychosocial Outcomes in Breast Reconstruction: Two-Year Postoperative Results from the Michigan Breast Reconstruction Outcomes Study," *Annals of Surgery* 247, no. 6 (2008): 1019–28. doi:10.1097/SLA.0b013e3181728a5c.

7. Lautner et al., "Disparities in the Use of Breast-Conserving Therapy Among Patients with Early-Stage Breast Cancer."

CHAPTER 3: MASTECTOMY: WHAT TO EXPECT

1. Angelina Jolie, "My Medical Choice," *New York Times*, May 14, 2013. http://www.nytimes.com/2013/05/14/opinion/my-medical-choice.html?_r=0.

2. National Cancer Institute, http://www.cancer.gov/types/breast/risk-reducing-surgery-fact-sheet.

3. http://www.breastcancer.org/research-news/more-choosing-mx-over-lx.

CHAPTER 4: A VETERAN'S STORY: LUMPECTOMY

1. K. Zhu et al., "Cancer Incidence in the U.S. Military Population: Comparison with Rates from the SEER Program," *Cancer Epidemiology, Biomarkers and Prevention* 18, no. 6 (2009), 1740–45.

2. Armed Forces Health Surveillance Center, "Incident Diagnoses of Cancers and Cancer-Related Deaths, Active Component, U.S. Armed Forces 2000–2011," *MSMR* 19, no. 6 (June 2012).

CHAPTER 5: RECONSTRUCTION WITH TISSUE

1. American Society of Plastic Surgeons, http://www.plasticsurgery.org/news/plastic-surgery-statistics/2014-statistics.html.

2. Oscar Ochoa et al., "Abdominal Wall Stability and Flap Complications After Deep Inferior Epigastric Breast Reconstruction: Does Body Mass Index Make a Difference? Analysis of 418 Patients and 639 Flaps," *Plastic and Reconstructive Surgery* 130, no. 1 (2012): 21e–33e, http://journals.lww.com/plasreconsurg/Fulltext/2012/07000/Abdominal_Wall_Stability_and_Flap_Complications.9.aspx.

CHAPTER 6: MEDICAL DESTINATIONS

1. Frank DellaCroce et al., "Nipple-Sparing Mastectomy and Ptosis: Perforator Flap Breast Reconstruction Allows Full Secondary Mastopexy with Complete Nipple Areolar Repositioning," *Plastic Reconstructive Surgery* 136, no. 1 (2015): 1e–9e. doi:10.1097/PRS.0000000000001325.

CHAPTER 7: SILICONE IMPLANTS

1. U.S. Food and Drug Administration, "Regulatory History of Breast Implants in the U.S.," http://www.fda.gov/MedicalDevices/ProductsandMedicalProcedures/ImplantsandProsthetics/BreastImplants/ucm064461.htm.

2. American Society of Plastic Surgeons, http://www.plasticsurgery.org/news/plastic-surgery-statistics/2014-statistics.html.

3. BreastCancer.org, http://www.breastcancer.org/treatment/surgery/reconstruction/types/implants.

4. Sheila Biggs, email to author, member-only data, American Society of Plastic Surgeons, June 26, 2015.

5. U.S. Food and Drug Administration, "Labeling of Approved Breast Implants," product inserts, http://www.fda.gov/MedicalDevices/ProductsandMedicalProcedures/ImplantsandProsthetics/BreastImplants/ucm063743.htm.

CHAPTER 8: SALINE IMPLANTS

1. http://www.plasticsurgery.org/news/plastic-surgery-statistics/2014-statistics.html.

2. Mentor Worldwide LLC, http://www.mentorwwllc.com/global-us/ProductInformation.aspx.

3. http://www.mentorwwllc.com/global-us/ProductInformation.aspx.

CHAPTER 9: FLAT OR ONE-BREASTED

1. https://www.youtube.com/watch?v=zMk8pj4TR64.

CHAPTER 10: UNEVEN RESULTS

1. Dunya Atisha et al., "Prospective Analysis of Long-Term Psychosocial Outcomes in Breast Reconstruction: Two-Year Postoperative Results from the Michigan Breast Reconstruction Outcomes Study," *Annuals of Surgery* 247, no. 6 (2008): 1019–28.

CHAPTER 11: DELAYED RECONSTRUCTION

1. Sheila Biggs, email to author, member-only data, American Society of Plastic Surgeons, June 26, 2015.
2. www.plasticsurgery.org.
3. http://brava.com.

CHAPTER 12: THE NIPPLE: THE ULTIMATE CHALLENGE

1. vinniemyers.com.

CHAPTER 13: REVISIONISTS

1. American Society of Breast Surgeons, "Breast Reconstruction Typically a Multi-Step Process," April 30, 2015, https://www.breastsurgeons.org/docs2015/press/PMBR%20-%20Roberts%20-%20ASBrS%2015%20Press%20Release.pdf.
2. http://www.breastimplantsafety.org/PatientswithImplants/index.php.
3. Scott Spear, "Applications of Acellular Dermal Matrix in Revision Breast Cancer Surgery," *Plastic & Reconstructive Surgery* 133, no. 1 (2014): 1–10. doi:10.1097/01.prs.0000436810.88659.36
4. Lee Martin et al., "Acellular Dermal Matrix (ADM) Assisted Breast Reconstruction Procedures: Joint Guidelines from the Association of Plastic Surgery and the British Association of Plastic, Reconstructive and Aesthetic Surgeons," *European Journal of Surgical Oncology* 39, no. 5 (2013).

CHAPTER 15: LYMPHEDEMA

1. Curtis Whitehair and Eric Wisotzky, *Managing Breast Cancer* (Washington: MedStar NRH Press, 2014).

CHAPTER 16: ARAB CULTURE

1. Suzanne Mellon et al., "Knowledge, Attitudes and Beliefs of Arab-American Women Regarding Inherited Cancer Risk," *Journal of Genetic Counseling* 22, no. 2 (2013): 268–76. doi:10/1007/s10897-012-9546-2.
2. Myriad Genetics, Prevalence Table, http://d1izdzz43r5o67.cloudfront.net/brac/BART-table-faq.pdf.

CHAPTER 20: PREVIVORS

1. Ananias Diokno and Patricia Anstett, *Triumph: Inspirational Stories from Beaumont* (Royal Oak, MI: Beaumont Health System, 2014).

CHAPTER 22: PREGNANCY

1. Elyce Cardonick et al., "Development of Children Born to Mothers with Cancer During Pregnancy: Comparing In Utero Chemotherapy-Exposed Children with Non-Exposed Controls," *American Journal of Obstetrics and Gynecology* 212, no. 5 (2014): 658.

2. National Cancer Institute, http://www.cancer.gov/types/breast/hp/pregnancy-breast-treatment-pdq.

Glossary

COMMON TERMS, EXPLAINED IN CONTEXT OF BREAST SURGERY

acelullar dermal matrix. Abbreviated as ADM, these are products made of sterilized human and animal collagen used in breast reconstruction to add support or shape.

adhesive capsulitis. Shoulder stiffness or pain, or frozen shoulder. See also **postmastectomy pain syndrome**.

adjuvant therapy. Chemotherapy, radiation, and other therapies given after surgery to lower the risk of cancer recurrence. See also **delayed breast reconstruction**.

anatomically shaped implant. One of several terms to describe a harder gel substance used in newer silicone breast implants and designed to more closely resemble a natural breast. See also **cohesive implants, gummy bear implants**.

areola. Pigmented skin around the nipple.

aromatase inhibitors. Drugs such as exemestane that block the production of estrogen by the body.

autologous breast reconstruction. One of several methods to build a breast with tissue, fat, blood vessels, and sometimes muscle from the abdomen, thigh, butt, or back.

axilla. Armpit.

axillary dissection. Incision in the underarm area to remove several or more lymph nodes to determine whether they contain cancer. Cancer that has spread to these lymph nodes is more likely to recur. See also lymph node dissection; **sentinel lymph node biopsy**.

brachytherapy. Internal radiation. See also **radiation therapy**.

BRCA1 and BRCA2. Genes that suppress or prevent cancer. When there is a mutation in a BRCA1 or BRCA2 gene, an individual has increased cancer risk.

breast augmentation. Elective breast procedures for cosmetic purposes. Also called **augmentation mammoplasty**.

217

breast lift. Surgery, known as mastopexy, to lift and shape a breast. It often is done in a second "touch up" procedure after mastectomy and breast reconstruction.

cancer staging. System to identify cancer by tumor characteristics and metastasis. In breast cancer, it refers to the size of the tumor and whether it is in the breast only or has spread to nearby lymph nodes or other places in the body. Larger tumors (especially those that are more than five centimeters—about two inches—in diameter) are more likely to recur than small tumors. Breast cancer often first spreads to the lymph nodes under the arm (axillary lymph nodes). During surgery, doctors usually remove some of these underarm lymph nodes to determine whether they contain cancer cells. Cancer that has spread to these lymph nodes is more likely to recur.

capsular contracture. A complication of breast implant reconstruction when scar tissue forms around the implant, tightens it, and makes it hard, firm, and sometimes painful.

closed capsulotomy. Technique used to relieve capsular contracture involving manually squeezing the breast to break the hard capsule around an implant.

cohesive implant. One of several terms to describe a harder substance used in newer breast implants. Also called anatomical or gummy bear implants, they are designed to more closely resemble a natural breast.

contralateral prophylactic mastectomy. Removal of the opposite, non-cancerous breast.

cording. Development of a ropelike structure under or down the arm, more common after radiation or surgery with lymph node dissection. Also called axillary web syndrome. See also **lymphedema**.

deep vein thrombosis. A surgery complication that causes the development of a blood clot, or thrombus, in one or more of the deep veins in the body, often the legs.

delayed breast reconstruction. Breast reconstruction performed months or years after mastectomy, often to allow women to have chemotherapy or radiation. See also **adjuvant therapy**.

DIEP flap. Deep Inferior Epigastric Perforator flap is a breast reconstruction procedure that takes tissue and blood vessels from the abdomen to create a new breast.

direct-to-implant breast reconstruction. In what doctors also call one-step implant reconstruction, implants are placed in the chest at the time of mastectomy, avoiding the use of temporary expanders. See also **expander**.

donor site. The area where a surgeon harvests skin, blood, fat, and sometimes muscle from one area of the body, the donor site, and moves it to the chest to create a breast.

drains. Temporary tubes inserted after mastectomy and reconstruction surgery to remove chest fluids and prevent the buildup of blood clots at incision sites.

expander. A temporary implant with a metal port through which saline water is inserted at intervals over three or four months to stretch the chest skin and muscle to hold a breast implant. It is replaced with a permanent implant.

fat-grafting. A liposuction technique used in breast reconstruction that takes fat from other parts of the body that is sterilized and injected into the breasts for support and contours around an implant or flap.

flaps. Skin, fat, blood vessels, and sometimes muscle used to reconstruct a breast. See also **autologous breast reconstruction**.

GAP flap. Breast reconstruction using the Superior Gluteal Artery Perforator tissue and blood supply from the buttocks. Sometimes referred to as S-GAP. See also **autologous breast reconstruction**.

gene. A sequence of deoxyribonucleic acid (DNA) and ribonucleic acid (RNA) that contains the heredity of a living organism.

gummy bear implants. See anatomically shaped **breast implants**.

hematoma. Blood pooling beneath the skin.

hormone receptor status. The cells of many breast tumors express receptors for the hormones estrogen and progesterone. Tumors with cells that do not express hormone receptors are more likely to recur. Doctors can determine whether a tumor expresses hormone receptors with laboratory tests.

HER2 status. Tumors that produce too much of a protein called HER2 are more likely to recur. Doctors can determine whether a tumor produces too much HER2 with a laboratory test.

hysterectomy. Surgical removal of the uterus, with or without other nearby organs and tissue. In a total hysterectomy, the uterus and cervix are removed. In a radical hysterectomy, the uterus, cervix, both ovaries, both fallopian tubes and nearby tissue are removed. In a radical hysterectomy, the uterus, cervix, both ovaries, both fallopian tubes and nearby tissue are removed. In a total hystectomy with salpingo-oophorectomy, the uterus and one of both ovaries and tubes are removed.

IGAP flap. Breast reconstruction with an Inferior Gluteal Artery Perforator flap, using skin, fat, tissue, and blood supply from the buttocks. See also **tissue-based breast reconstruction**.

inframammary fold. The crease under the breast, and a common incision site.

Latissimus Dorsi flap. A surgical technique that takes a flap of tissue, muscle, fat, blood supply, and skin from a woman's back to make a new breast. It is tunneled under the skin and attached to its donor site, leaving the blood supply intact. See also **autologous breast reconstruction**.

lollipop incision. One of several popular incisions in which surgeons open a wedge of triangular tissue under the breast and around the nipple and areola.

lumpectomy. A surgical procedure to remove a lump or area of concern and a small amount of normal tissue around it.

lymphatic drainage. Methods such as massage that move along fluids associated with lymphedema from swollen areas of the body.

lymphatic system. A weblike system that filters body fluids. It has muscles and a one-way valve system that help move fluid in the right direction.

lymphedema. Chronic pain and swelling in the arm, breast, chest wall, or neck, caused by surgery, lymph node dissection, radiation, or cancer itself. It occurs when the body's lymphatic system, a backup network to the circulatory and immune systems that traps bacteria and other germs, is injured and fluids back up within the lymphatic fluid. It causes pain and swelling in the arm, breast, chest wall, or neck. It can be detected with a test known as lymphoscintigraphy. See also **lymph node dissection.**

lymph node dissection. Surgical removal of one or more lymph nodes to check if cancer has spread beyond the breast.

lymph nodes. Bean-shaped structures found throughout the body, including the chest, under the arm, or axilla, and above the collarbone. See also **axilla, lymph node dissection**.

Mamma Print. Test that helps predict whether stage 1 or stage 2 breast cancer that is node-negative will spread to other parts of the body. If the risk of the cancer spreading is high, chemotherapy may be given to lower the risk.

mastectomy. Surgical removal of the breast to treat or prevent cancer.

mastopexy. See **breast lift**.

medical oncologist. Medical doctor specializing in chemotherapy.

metastasis. Spread of cancer from the original site to another organ.

neoadjuvant therapy. Chemotherapy or radiation delivered at the beginning of treatment, prior to surgery. See also **delayed breast reconstruction**.

Oncotype DX. Test that helps select patients who will best benefit from chemotherapy during or after treatment. It is for women with stage 1 or 2 breast cancer and tumors that are estrogen-receptor positive and node-negative. See also **cancer staging**.

PAP flap. An autologous breast reconstruction procedure using tissue from the back of the upper thigh.

partial mastectomy. Surgical procedure to remove part of the breast that contains cancer and some normal tissue around it. Some lymph nodes under the arm also may be removed for biopsy. See also **segmental mastectomy**.

physiatrist. Medical doctor specializing in rehabilitation medicine and management of post-surgery issues.

postmastectomy pain syndrome. A type of chronic pain disorder that can occur following breast cancer procedures, particularly those operations that remove tissue in the upper outer quadrant of the breast or axilla.

prophylactic mastectomy. Operation to remove one or both breasts to reduce the risk of breast cancer. The term refers to surgery for women with breast cancer who choose to remove a non-cancerous breast as well as preventive procedures.

prothesis. A form made of various materials to supplant or fill out the breast in women after lumpectomy or mastectomy.

quadrantectomy. See **segmental mastectomy**.

radiation oncologist. Medical doctor specializing in radiation therapy.

radiation therapy. Cancer treatment that uses high-energy x-rays or other types of radiation to kill cancer cells. External radiation therapy uses a machine outside the body to send radiation toward the cancer. Internal radiation therapy or brachytherapy uses a radioactive substance placed inside needles, seeds, wires, or catheters that are placed directly into or near the cancer.

salpingo-oophorectomy. Surgery to remove ovaries and fallopian tubes, for ovarian cancer or to prevent it.

segmental mastectomy. Also called partial mastectomy or quadrantectomy. Surgery that removes up to one-quarter of the breast, more tissue than a lumpectomy. See also **lumpectomy.**

sentinel lymph node biopsy. The first of several lymph nodes removed and analyzed as an indicator of a cancer's invasion into other tissue beyond the breast. See also **axillary dissection; lymph node dissection.**

seroma. An accumulation of fluid.

SIEA flap. An autologous breast reconstruction procedure much like a DIEP flap using abdominal tissue and the superficial inferior epigastric artery and perforator veins.

tamoxifen. Federally approved drug, typically taken for five years after breast surgery, to reduce the recurrence of cancer in women who have a five-year risk of developing breast cancer. It blocks estrogen, inhibiting the growth of some breast cancers fueled by the hormone. It is approved for both premenopausal and postmenopausal women.

tissue-based breast reconstruction. See **autologous breast reconstruction.**

TRAM flap. Also known as Transverse Rectus Abdominus Musculocutaneous flap. Reconstruction with abdominal fat, along with nearby muscle and blood vessels. See also **autologous breast reconstruction**.

TUG flap. Breast reconstruction using the Transverse Upper Gracilis perforator flap. Breast reconstruction using muscle and fat from along the bottom fold of the buttock, extending to the inner thigh. See also **autologous breast reconstruction**.

tumor grade. Method using a microscope to analyze how closely tumor cells resemble normal breast cells. Tumors with cells that bear little or no resemblance to normal breast cells are called *poorly differentiated tumors* and are more likely to recur. Women with tumor cells that look like normal breast cells, or well-differentiated tumors, tend to have a better prognosis. See also **cancer staging**.

unilateral mastectomy. A single mastectomy; removal of the cancerous breast only.

Sources: National Cancer Institute; U.S. Food and Drug Administration; American Society of Plastic Surgeons; National Lymphedema Network; PRMA Plastic Surgery, San Antonio, TX.

Bibliography

American Society of Breast Surgeons. "Breast Reconstruction Typically a Multi-Step Process." April 30, 2015. https://www.breastsurgeons.org/docs2015/press/PMBR%20-%20Roberts%20-%20ASBrS%2015%20Press%20Release.pdf.

American Society of Plastic Surgeons. 2014 Plastic Surgery Statistics. http://www.plasticsurgery.org/news/plastic-surgery-statistics/2014-statistics.html.

American Society of Plastic Surgeons. "Tattoo Artists Play New Role in Breast Reconstruction." http://ww.plasticsurgery.org/news/tattoo-artists-play-new-role-in-breast-reconstruction.html.

Diokno, Ananias, and Patricia Anstett. *Triumph: Inspirational Stories from Beaumont*. Royal Oak, MI: Beaumont Health System, 2014, 85–102.

Fitzgerald, Judith Medeiros. *A Teacher's Journey . . . What Breast Cancer Taught Me*. CreateSpace Independent Publishing Platform, 2012.

Friedman, Sue, Rebecca Sutphen, and Kathy Steligo. *Confronting Hereditary Breast and Ovarian Cancer*. Baltimore: Johns Hopkins Press Health Book, 2012.

Jolie, Angelina, "My Medical Choice," *New York Times*, May 14, 2013. http://www.nytimes.com/2013/05/14/opinion/my-medical-choice.html?_r=0.

Lautner, Meeghan, et al. "Disparities in the Use of Breast-Conserving Therapy Among Patients with Early-Stage Breast Cancer." *JAMA Surgery*, July 17, 2005. http://archsurg.jamanetwork.com/article.aspx?articleid=2322835.

Love, Susan M., and Karen Lindsey. *Dr. Susan Love's Breast Book*. Boston: Merloyd Lawrence, 2015.

Mentor Worldwide LLC. http://www.mentorwwllc.com/global-us/ProductInformation.aspx.

Morrow, Monica, et al. "Access to Breast Reconstruction after Mastectomy and Patient Perspectives on Reconstruction Decision Making." *JAMA Surgery* 149 no. 10 (2014): 1015–21.

Myers, Vinnie. Vinniemyers.com.

Narod, Steven, Javaid Iqbal, Vasily Giannakeas, Victoria Sopik, and Ping Sun. "Breast Cancer Mortality After a Diagnosis of Ductal Carcinoma in Situ." *JAMA Oncology* 1, no. 7 (2015), 888–96. http://oncology.jamanetwork.com/article.aspx?articleid=2427491.

National Cancer Institute. http://www.cancer.gov/types/breast/risk-reducing-surgery-fact-sheet.

National Cancer Institute. Breast Cancer Treatment and Pregnancy—for Health Professionals. http://www.cancer.gov/types/breast/hp/pregnancy-breast-treatment-pdq.

National Comprehensive Cancer Network guidelines. Stages I and II Breast Cancer. http://www.nccn.org/patients/guidelines/stage_i_ii_breast/index.html.

National Institutes of Health, Consensus Development Conference Statement. https://consensus.nih.gov/1990/1990earlystagebreastcancer081html.htm.

SSSO-ASTRO Consensus Guideline. "Margins for Breast-Conserving Surgery with Whole Breast Irradiation in Stage I and II Invasive Breast Cancer." http://www.surgonc.org/docs/default-source/pdf/sso-astro_consensus_guideline_on_margins_for_breast_conserving_surgery_final.pdf?sfvrsn=2.

Steligo, Kathy. *The Breast Reconstruction Book*, Third Edition. Baltimore: Johns Hopkins University Press, 2012.

U.S. Department of Labor. "Your Rights After a Mastectomy." www.dol.gov/ebsa/Publications/whcra.html.

U.S. Food and Drug Administration. "Regulatory History of Breast Implants in the U.S." http://www.fda.gov/MedicalDevices/ProductsandMedicalProcedures/ImplantsandProsthetics/BreastImplants/ucm064461.htm.

Whitehair, Curtis, and Eric Wisotzky. *Managing Breast Cancer*. Washington: MedStar NRH Press, 2014.

Index

acellular dermal matrix (ADM), 3, 25–26, 64, 123–24. *See also* breast revision
Aburabia, Majd, 146, 151–52
ACCESS, 146–47, 153–54
Adams, Betti, 93–95
Ali, Haythem, 152–53, 202
American Academy on Communications in Healthcare, 175
arab culture, 145–54
Ashikari, Andrew, 21, 66
autologous breast reconstruction, 37–49; average hospital stay, 48; DIEP flap, 37, 39, 41–43, 48–49, 52–59; IGAP/SGAP flap, 42; latissimusi dorsi flap, 42–43; PAP flap, 42; recovery after, 48–49; statistics, 38, 43; SIEA flap, 38, 42–43, 47–48; TRAM flap, 39, 41–44, 53; TUG flap, 42; types of incisions, 39, 46. *See also* health insurance
Aziz, Ghada, 147–50

Becker, Hilton, 63
Blain, Sharon Fitzpatrick, 86–89
Blum, Craig, 55
Brava device, 108–109
BRCA genes: defined, 178; founder genes, 181; national surveillance guidelines, 189; risk reduction benefits of preventive surgeries, 179; testing issues, 190–96. *See also* health insurance

breast cancer: early-stage, 4, 10, 12; incidence, 4; national guidelines, 17; during pregnancy, 202–206; triple-negative, 1–2; vaccine, 5
breast forms, 162–65
breast implants, saline, 25, 63, 65, 73–77, 180
breast implants, silicone, 61–72; anatomical, 25, 68–69; capsular contracture from, 68; cohesive gel (*see* breast implants, anatomical); complications, 67, 119–26; direct-to-implant, 64–67; distortion, 63; gummy-bear (*see* cohesive gel implants); expanders, 3–6, 25–26; federal silicone moratorium, 10, 62, 74; federal warnings, 67; issues for large-framed, busty women, 3; rupture, removal, 67
breast lift: as second stage of breast reconstruction, 21, 46, 49, 57–58. *See also* breast revision
breast reconstruction: anesthesia, 23; changing demographics, 2, 177–78; complications, 48; delayed, 101–10; going without, 79–91; federal laws about, 4, 190; high-volume centers, 48, 52; impact on sex, intimacy, 127–34; mental health impact, 13–14; preventive surgery, 2, 4, 177–85; reasons women decline, 4; recovery, 13, 27–28, 58, 209; resources, 210; uneven results, 93–99. *See* also autologous breast

reconstruction; breast implants, saline; breast implants, silicone; health insurance
breast revision, 119–26; as a second stage of reconstruction, 21, 45–46; high-volume practices, 48, 52, 119; increase with introduction of fat-grafting, 120; reasons for, 120–21

Cancer Prevention and Treatment Fund, 11
Carpenter, Michele, 20, 23–25
Castellenos, Maria Cruz, 96–97
Chaiyasate Kongrit, 43, 105–106, 168–69
Chrysopoulo, Minas, 39, 43, 107
cohesive gel implants. *See* breast implants, silicone, anatomical
Colwell, Amy, 21
Conley, Jill, 90–91
contralateral double mastectomy. *See* mastectomy, contralateral double
cording, 140. *See* lymphedema
Courson, Jill, 6–7
Coutee, Terri, 106
Cox, Belinda, 64, 167, 169

Dauphinais, Donna, 111–17, 119–26
Dekhne, Nayana, 180
Disa, Joseph, 40, 65, 121
doctors: assembling a team, 207–208; hospital referral patterns, 168–69; insurance network restrictions, 167; questions to ask, 16, 18; resources to find one, 168, 172
ductal carcinoma in situ (DCIS). *See* breast cancer, early stage

Elkus, Robert, 31
Erzen, Sara, 3, 201–206
expanders. *See* breast implants, silicone; breast implants, saline

Facing Our Risk Empowered, (FORCE), 21–22, 63, 188–89
fat-grafting, 3, 49, 120, 123. *See* breast revision
Fitzgerald, Judith Medeiros, 5–6

Flat & Fabulous, 79
flat-chested, one-breasted, 79–91
Flat Friends, 79
Fonfa, Ann, 79–83
Ford Motor Co. Warriors in Pink, 7
Friedman, Sue, 179

Galligan, Kathleen, 29–35
Goldberg, Sandy, 160–61
Gorosh, Marla Rowe, 175
Gow, Rose, 97–99, 128
gummy bear implants. *See* breast implants, silicone, anatomical

Hacker, Marjorie, 34, 73–77
Hamade, Hiam, 145–47, 153
Hammad, Adnan, 153–54
Hammond, Dennis, 68, 119, 122–26
Havorson, Eric, 112
Hayes, Daniel, 112
health insurance: federal requirements about genetic counseling and preventive surgery in high-risk women, 4, 190; federal coverage requirements for breast forms or reconstruction after mastectomy, 3; network limits on doctor selection, 167; state laws, 158
Heck, Sharon Kiley, 9, 15–16
Hernandez, Ivy, 187–88, 197–99
Hope for Two: The Pregnant with Cancer Network, 203
Horton, Karen, 74–75, 119–20, 122

Johnson, Linda Jo, 163–66
Johnston, Joe, 45
Jolie, Angelina, 2, 179–80

Karlan, Scott, 21
Kreifels, Jill, 121–22
Kronowitz, Steven, 64, 102, 104

Land, Kim, 37–49
Lazarovitz, Karen, 180–83
Ley, Michele, 106
Lichter, Allen, 11
Littleton, Johanna, 80, 83

liposuction. *See* fat-grafting
lumpectomy, 29–35; factors
  influencing choice, 14; national
  consensus guidelines, 4–5; reasons
  women decline, 4; reexicision rates,
  5; statistics, 4; survival compared to
  mastectomy, 4, 11; tumor margins,
  5. *See also* radiation
lymphedema, 137–43
lymphoscintigraphy, 139

MacDonald, Molly, 155–157. *See also*
  The Pink Fund
Mapes, Diane, 108–10, 128
mastectomy, 19–28; anesthesia, 23;
  changing patient demographics,
  2; contralateral double, 4,
  10–12; double prophylactic, 2, 4,
  10–11, 20, 38, 79, 116–18; factors
  influencing choice, 4, 14; federal,
  state laws affecting coverage, 3,
  158; guidelines on prophylactic
  mastectomy, 11; long-term
  studies of, 13, 94; mental health
  issues, 13–14; nipple-sparing,
  2, 20–21, 24, 52–54, 58; postmastectomy pain syndrome,
  137–38; robotic, 103–104; statistics,
  13; types of, 22; recovery after, 28;
  resources, 17. *See also* autologous
  breast reconstruction; breast
  implants, silicone; breast implants,
  saline
Medaglia, Guy, 161
Meininger, Michael, 15, 68, 113–14,
  116–17, 132
Michigan Reconstruction Outcomes
  Consortium, 13, 94
Mitchell, Kimberlee, 103–104
Momoh, Adeyiza, 40
Morang, Julie, 172–75
Morrow, Monica, 4
Musser, Barbara, 129–36
Myers, Vinnie, 111–15
My Hope Chest, 157–59
Newman, Lisa, 12
nipples, 111–18: injectable fillers
  used, 116–17; loss of sensation

after reconstruction, 67; surgical
  reconstruction of, 112; tattoos,
  111–13

Palmer, Natalie, 89–90
Perkins, Cheryl, 1–2, 7–8
The Pink Fund, 7, 117, 155–56
preimplantation genetic diagnosis, 184
previvor, 179

radiation: complications, 7, 10,
  33; factors influencing choice,
  14; factors leading to delayed
  reconstruction, 101–104
Rickert, Emmy Pontz, 61–72
Rojas, Alejandra, 3, 19, 188–96
Rojas, Socorro, 188–89
Rojas, Veronica Gudino, 19, 119–26,
  157–60, 188–89
Rothe, Kelly, 177–80, 184–85
Rustom, Mohamad, 150–52

A Silver Lining Foundation, 160
Salzberg, Andrew, 64, 66
Santilli, Susan, 140–41
Savoretti, Alisa, 157–60
Schwarz, Karl, 182
Selber, Jesse, 68, 101
sentinel lymph node biopsy, 24, 46
sex, 127–36
Shah, Forum, 189–96
Sheffield, Sharon, 137–41
Simon, Susan, 105
Stollier, Allan, 55
Spear, Scott, 63
Spectrum implant. *See* breast implants,
  saline
Studvent, Donald, 128–33
Studvent, Katrina, 128–33
Sullivan, Scott, 52–53
Swift, Mikeal, 58–59

tamoxifen, 31
tattoos. *See* nipples
Taylor, Linda Jo, 163–66
Thompson, Elizabeth, 66–67
Turpin, Ivan, 23, 25–28
Trahan, Chris, 56

vascularized lymph node transfer, 143.
    See lymphedema

Weaver, Ty, 156–57
Weinraub, Erika Rojas, 188, 196
Wilkins, Edwin, 13, 69

Wise, Whit, 53
Wisotzky, Eric, 141–43

Zakalik, Dana, 179
Zuckerman, Diana, 11, 14, 69

About the Author and Photographer

Patricia Anstett is an experienced medical writer who worked for forty years in newspaper journalism in Chicago, Washington, D.C., and Detroit, her hometown. For the last twenty-two years of her professional newspaper career she was a medical writer for the *Detroit Free Press*, retiring in 2011. Her award-winning stories covered various aspects of breast cancer and breast implant surgery. The American Society of Plastic Surgeons honored her work in 1995 with an unsolicited national award. The year before, she also received the Vivian Castleberry Award, a national competition honoring top reporting on women's issues, for her coverage of new breast biopsy options. The American Cancer Society and the Barbara Karmanos Cancer Institute each have given her awards for the accuracy and comprehensiveness of her breast cancer reporting. Anstett's reporting has won national, state, and local awards for breaking news, beat, and feature writing. She has been honored as Journalist of the Year, Detroit chapter, Society of Professional Journalists, and received the top Headliner award from the Detroit chapter of the Association of Women in Communications. Her freelance articles have appeared in *Reader's Digest*, the *National Observer*, the *Chicago Tribune*, *Washingtonian* magazine, and *Paris Match*. She was part of a reporting team that published *The Suicide Machine* about the first forty-seven patients to seek help from the late Dr. Jack Kevorkian. She is married and the mother of three children.

Kathleen Galligan, photographer, is an Emmy award–winning photographer and videographer who specializes in women's health, social justice, mental health, poverty, and juvenile justice issues. A single mother with two sons, Galligan worked as a plastic surgery center photographer before joining the *Detroit Free Press* in 2002. Her first online documentary project, *Christ Child*, about a residential treatment center for severely abused and neglected boys, was awarded a national news and documentary Emmy in 2009. Her work also has captured a National Headliners Award in journalistic innovation as well as numerous national and state awards in photography.

229